The Institute of Biology's
Studies in Biology no. 164

The Human Skin

E. J. Wood

M.A., D.Phil.
Senior Lecturer,
Department of Biochemistry,
University of Leeds

P. T. Bladon

B.Sc., Ph.D., M.I.Biol.
Research Fellow,
Leeds Dermatological Research Foundation,
Department of Dermatology,
The General Infirmary at Leeds

Edward Arnold

© E. J. Wood and P. T. Bladon 1985

First published in Great Britain 1985
by Edward Arnold (Publishers) Ltd
41 Bedford Square, London WC1B 3DQ

Edward Arnold (Australia) Pty Ltd
80 Waverley Road
Caulfield East
Victoria 3145
Australia

Edward Arnold
3 East Read Street
Baltimore
Maryland 21201
U.S.A

British Library Cataloguing in Publication Data

Wood, E.J.
  The human skin.—(The Institute of Biology's
  studies in biology, ISSN 0537-9024; no. 164)
  1. Skin
  I. Title   II. Bladon, P.T.   III. Series
  612'.79   QP88.5

  ISBN 0-7131-2900-X

Text set in 9/11pt Times
by The Castlefield Press
Printed and bound in Great Britain by Camelot Press

General Preface to the Series

Because it is no longer possible for one textbook to cover the whole field of biology while remaining sufficiently up to date, the Institute of Biology proposed this series so that teachers and students can learn about significant developments. The enthusiastic acceptance of 'Studies in Biology' shows that the books are providing authoritative views of biological topics.

The features of the series include the attention given to methods, the selected list of books for further reading and, wherever possible, suggestions for practical work.

Readers' comments will be welcomed by the Institute.

1985

Institute of Biology
20 Queensberry Place
London SW7 2DZ

Preface

The skin is an organ of great interest to biologists, biochemists and clinicians, but there are few books that deal at the rather basic level with skin from all of these aspects. The present book was written with the aim of introducing the biology, the biochemistry and some facets of skin diseases to the student. Recently there have been a number of very important developments in skin biochemistry research as well as in the medical treatment of skin disorders, not least the introduction of certain vitamin A derivatives or retinoids. In addition, knowledge is increasing in the area of the cell biology of wound-healing and melanogenesis, and of the processes involved in inflammation, skin immunology and allergies.

We hope that most students will find at least some of this of interest as part of their studies in biology, and that it will also satisfy or stimulate their curiosity about the marvellous organ that envelopes us all, and make them want to read further.

1985

E.J.W.
P.T.B.

Contents

General Preface to the Series   iii

Preface   iii

1   Introduction   1
1.1 Structure of skin   1.2 The glands of the skin
1.3 Innervation   1.4 Blood supply   1.5 Skin colour   1.6 The
flora and fauna of the skin

2   The Epidermis   6
2.1 Structure   2.2 The keratins   2.3 Keratinization
2.4 Keratohyaline granules   2.5 Terminal differentiation
2.6 The role of lipids   2.7 The sebaceous gland   2.8 Hair
2.9 Nails   2.10 Dermatoglyphics

3   The Dermis   20
3.1 Introduction   3.2 The function of the dermis
3.3 Collagen   3.4 Elastin   3.5 The ground substance
3.6 Dermal cells   3.7 Changes with ageing   3.8 Dermal
appendages   3.9 Blood supply and temperature control
3.10 Sweat glands   3.11 Innervation

4   Melanogenesis   32
4.1 Introduction   4.2 Melanocytes   4.3 Melanogenesis
4.4 Albinism   4.5 Melanocyte-stimulating hormone (MSH)
4.6 Suntan   4.7 Ultraviolet radiation   4.8 Sunlight induces
cancer   4.9 Freckles   4.10 Porphyria

5   Inflammation, Skin Immunology and Wound Healing   41
5.1 Introduction   5.2 Inflammation   5.3 Changes taking
place in inflammation   5.4 The immune system   5.5 IgE and
mast cells   5.6 Hypersensitivity   5.7 Hypersensitivity
mediated by immune complexes   5.8 Delayed hypersensitivity
5.9 Dermatitis   5.10 Drug reactions   5.11 Viruses and the
skin   5.12 Transplantation immunity   5.13 Wound healing
5.14 Hypertrophic scars and keloids

6   Diseases of the Skin   56
6.1 Introduction   6.2 Infections   6.3 Diseases of the
epidermis – acne   6.4 Eczema   6.5 Psoriasis   6.6 Diseases
of the dermis – the collagen diseases   6.7 Diseases of
collagen biosynthesis   6.8 Cancers of the skin   6.9 Basal
cell carcinoma   6.10 Squamous cell carcimona   6.11 Malignant
melanoma

Further Reading   67

Index   68

1 Introduction

The entire surface of the human body is covered by a layer of skin which presents a tough but flexible barrier to the exterior. As well as its more obvious protective role against physical trauma, the skin has a number of other important functions which are related to its forming the interface between the organism and the external environment. Not only does it prevent harmful things getting into the body but also its impermeability restricts water loss. The skin plays a major role in temperature regulation, and, being rich in nerve endings, forms an extensive sensory surface. In addition, it provides protection against damage by light because of the presence of pigments (melanins) which absorb the harmful ultraviolet part of the spectrum. Skin also has a metabolic role in relation to light. The action of light on a precursor compound in the skin produces vitamin D which has a role in calcium and phosphate metabolism.

1.1 Structure of skin

The skin is one of the largest organs in the body, constituting approximately one-eighth of the weight of a normal individual (Table 1–1). Its attachment to the body varies, being loose over most of the trunk and joint flexures, but relatively tight over the palms of the hands and soles of the feet. The thickness also varies: thus the skin of the eyelids is very thin, whilst that of the callus areas (palms and soles) is much thicker. The epithelium of the skin is continuous with those of the digestive, respiratory and genito-urinary systems at their external orifices.

Two layers are easily recognizable.

(1) The outer *epidermis* is cellular and avascular, and in the human, is 0.06–0.1 mm thick in most regions, but tending to be thicker on the back and much thicker in callus areas. The epidermis arises from the embryonic

Table 1–1 Weight of the various tissues of a 65 kg human male.

Tissue	kg fresh weight
Skeletal muscle	30.0
Internal organs	7.3
Bone	9.0
Skin and subcutaneous tissue	7.8
Adipose tissue	4.0
Blood	5.5
Connective tissue	1.0
Tissue fluids	0.4

ectoderm and forms most of the cutaneous appendages including the sweat and sebaceous glands, and the hair and the nails.

(2) The lower connective tissue layer or *dermis*, is much thicker than the epidermis (2–4 mm) and arises from the embryonic mesoderm. It supports the cutaneous appendages (hair follicles, sebaceous and sweat glands) and contains blood vessels, lymphatics and nerves. The dermis consists of a dense felt-work of connective tissue in which bundles of collagen fibrils predominate, intermingled with a mesh of elastic tissue. In comparison with the epidermis, the dermis contains relatively few cells, mainly fibroblasts, mast cells and macrophages.

Beneath the dermis is a layer of loose connective tissue called the *hypodermis*, sometimes recognized as a third layer of the skin. Over most of the body it forms a layer of adipose tissue, which provides thermal insulation and mechanical protection and the fat represents an energy reserve. Figure 1–1 is a simplified diagram of human skin.

The epidermis consists of epithelial cells that grow in layers, the deepest cell layer resting on the dermis and attached to it by a basement membrane. Cells of the basal layer on the basement membrane continuously divide, the daughter cells moving outwards towards the surface. As they do so they undergo a series of changes resulting ultimately in their becoming packed with the inert protein, *keratin*, and eventually dying and forming the flattish, dry, horny cells of the *stratum corneum*. This layer of dead cells is inert and relatively impervious. The dead cells are constantly being sloughed off at the surface throughout the life of the individual. The stratum corneum tends to be covered with a thin layer of *sebum*, an oily, waxy material produced by the sebaceous glands, which keeps the dead cell layer flexible and water-resistant.

1.2   The glands of the skin

The dermis is rich in follicles and glands which, as mentioned above, are in fact epidermal structures produced as down-growths from the epidermis. Two types of gland occur, sebaceous glands and sweat glands. The sebaceous glands produce the oily, lubricant material sebum. Sweat glands are responsible for producing sweat. The evaporation of sweat causes cooling which contributes to the maintenance of body temperature. Mammary glands are also skin structures that evolved from sweat glands.

Hairs are produced from follicles which develop at about the third month of foetal life as small buds of epithelial cells. From these buds develop the hair matrix, the sebaceous glands and the apocrine glands (see p. 28). The hair shaft itself consists of dead keratinized material. Each hair has an errector muscle, under involuntary control, that can cause the hair to stand on end. In most mammals this is a method of 'thickening' the coat and preventing heat loss and often has other functions in frightening predators or in courtship displays. In humans where the hair, except on the head, genital regions and axillae, remains of the 'infantile' type its value in this respect is doubtful. Goose pimples are caused by the muscles pulling at the epidermis.

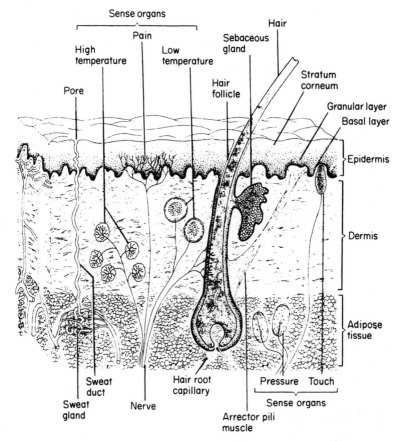

Fig. 1–1 Diagram to show the structure of human skin. (Reproduced from BECKETT, B.S. (1982)). *Biology – A Modern Introduction*, 2nd edition. Oxford University Press. © B.S. Beckett, 1982.)

1.3 Innervation

The skin is well supplied with nerves which are constantly sending information about the environment to the central nervous system. The sensory nerves have a variety of endings, many being naked, while others end in sensory cells. This presumably enables a range of 'sensations' to be detected, from very light touch to heavy pressure or pain, heat and cold, and vibrations. Some areas such as the finger tips are much richer in nerve endings and are consequently more sensitive, than other regions. This can be tested with a pair of dividers, asking an individual to say whether he detects a double or a single prick in different regions of the body. Sympathetic fibres accompany the cutaneous nerves and go to the sweat glands, the blood vessels and errector muscles of the hairs.

1.4   Blood supply

Arteries paired with veins enter the lowest region of the dermis to form the dermal network. These vessels are visible on the undersurface of skin after removal. From this network, vessels rise vertically to supply the mid-dermal network which supplies the follicles, and the sub-epidermal network which supplies the epidermis and also functions in heat regulation. Highly developed nervous control is exercised over the blood-flow to the skin, as this plays a major role in temperature regulation. The greatest control is exercised through the smallest arteries which have the highest proportion of muscle in their walls. Shunts provide a means of short-circuiting the capillary circulation in the dermis to prevent heat loss.

1.5   Skin colour

The normal colour of skin results from a mixture of red due to the haemoglobin of the blood in the capillaries, yellow due to substances related to the carotene pigments of plants in the subcutaneous fat and in the epidermis, and brown due to the pigment melanin. Obviously dilation of the capillaries increases the degree of redness and reduction of their diameter, or anaemia, reduces the degree of redness. Racial and ethnic differences of skin colour are related to the number, size, shape and distribution of the cytoplasmic organelles that contain melanin, called melanosomes. These are produced by pigment cells (melanocytes) and then transferred to surrounding epidermal cells (keratinocytes). Exposure to sunlight produces a darkening of the skin, or tan, and increased pigmentation can also be due to changes in hormonal status as in pregnancy.

1.6   The flora and fauna of the skin

Skin is quite a rich habitat for microorganisms, including bacteria and fungi, as well as for certain small arthropods. The presence of a microbial flora must be regarded as normal, and the organisms are prevented from invading deeper into the body by chemical factors such as lysozyme in the tears and saliva and by the gastric acidity. The constant shedding of cells from the stratum corneum also has a cleansing effect. Many bacteria live on the skin surface. Some are obligate anaerobes, and many are harboured in the sebaceous glands and hair follicles. Presumably these commensals play some part in denying pathogens the opportunity to colonize. However, the delicate ecological balance is easily upset by some types of antimicrobial therapy as well as the use of steroids and immunosuppresssive agents. For example, it is a common finding that the yeast-like fungus *Candida*, normally present on skin and mucous membranes, which is resistant to most antibiotics, will tend to undergo explosive growth and infect the oral, oesophageal and vaginal tracts leading to candidiasis, or thrush, if broad-spectrum antibiotic therapy is instituted.

The dry surface of the skin, with constant shedding of horny cells, is not in fact a very favourable habitat for pathogenic organisms. In contrast, damp skin folds (e.g. the axillae, and the skin web between the toes) and other moist areas such as skin beneath bandages, favour the growth of such organisms. These are typical sites for the growth of *Candida* and other fungi such as the one that causes athlete's foot (p. 57).

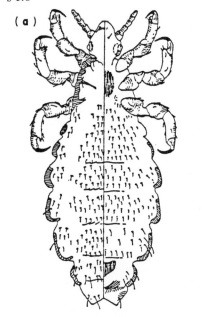

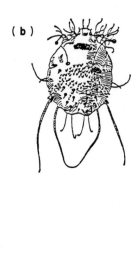

Fig. 1–2 Lice and scabies – arthropods that live on or in human skin. (a) Female body-louse (*Pediculus humanus*), left-dorsum, right venter, about 4 mm in length; (b) female scabies mite (*Sarcoptes scabiei*), length of body about 400 μm. (Reproduced from PASSMORE, R. and ROBSON, J.S. (Eds) (1970). *A Companion to Medical Studies*, Vol. 2, by courtesy of Blackwell Scientific Publications Ltd, Oxford.)

Several types of arthropod can inhabit the human skin. For example, the mite (Arachnida), *Demodex follicularum*, is cigar-shaped, about 0.3 mm long, and inhabits the ducts of the sebaceous glands, normally quite harmlessly. It is an obligate parasite and probably feeds on cellular debris and bacteria. After copulation has taken place at the orifice of the pilosebaceous follicle, the female deposits eggs in the sebaceous gland. The eggs hatch in 2–3 days, and after two nymphal stages, each lasting several days, the adult mite has a life-span of about 2 weeks. Head and body lice, *Pediculus capitis* and *Pediculus corporis*, have claws that enable them to grasp and hold on to hairs (Fig. 1–2a). These animals can only survive for a few hours away from a host and hence infection is mostly spread by personal contact. They feed by piercing the skin to draw blood. Infestation leads to irritation and scratching that may damage the skin and permit secondary infection. They can also transmit other diseases such as the Rickettsial epidemic typhus. *Sarcoptes scabiei* (Fig. 1–2b) causes scabies which again is transmitted mainly by direct contact. The mites live within the keratinized layers of the epidermis and the female burrows and lays eggs at intervals. Scabies mites are found mostly in the webs and sides of fingers, the fronts of the wrists, the nipples, umbilicus and genital regions. Such infestations are normally successfully treated by means of DDT, malathion or other insecticide, together with attention to cleanliness of the body and clothes.

2 The Epidermis

2.1 Structure

The epidermis, which is the most superficial layer of the skin, may be described as a keratinized stratified squamous epithelium. Several layers of cells may be recognized histologically. The very lowest layer, or *stratum basale*, sometimes called the *stratum germinativum*, consists of a single layer of more or less cylindrical cells with basophilic cytoplasm and centrally placed, elongated nuclei. These cells are joined to a basement membrane which marks the junction between epidermis and dermis. In vertical section this junction presents a wavy appearance (see Fig. 1–1 and p. 21) because of the dermal papillae. Cells are produced from the stratum basale by mitosis and these move outwards, i.e. to the exterior, gradually undergoing a process known as *keratinization*, finally to be shed from the surface as fully keratinized dead squamous cells or *squames*. A typical cell takes 2–3 weeks to pass from the stratum basale to the surface, and in the course of its journey it undergoes a number of transitions, leading to the characteristic histological appearance of the cells at each level.

Also found amongst the basal cells are the dendritic melanocytes. These have an independent lineage, being derived from the neural crest, and are responsible for skin pigmentation (p. 32). A third cell line making up the epidermal population is the Langerhans cell. This is also dendritic and is found in the granular layer, but is not related to the pigment system. The function and biological significance of these cells is unknown. For descriptive purposes the layers of epidermal cells moving outwards from the stratum basale are – *stratum spinosum; stratum granulosum; stratum lucidum;* and *stratum corneum* (Fig. 2–1). It should be stressed however that only in thick skin (e.g. plantar and palmar regions) are all five layers easily recognizable, but generally the 'spinous' cells and 'granular' cells can be recognized.

The *stratum spinosum* which lies immediately over the basal layer consists of 2–6 rows of polyhedral cells which tend to become more flattened as they move towards the surface. The name spinous cells was given because in the light microscope the cells appeared to be joined together by intercellular bridges giving individual cells a spiny appearance. It can be seen in the electron microscope that these bridges, called *desmosomes*, are in fact small areas of contact between cells. They correspond to points of attachment of bundles of filaments, called *tonofilaments*, to the plasma membrane of the cell. Tonofilaments are made of the insoluble fibrous protein, *keratin*. In fact similar filaments can also be observed in the basal layer cells.

Above the spiny cells is the *stratum granulosum* which consists of 1–3 layers of more or less diamond-shaped cells. These cells have darkly-staining nuclei and the cells appear to be packed with basophilic granules called

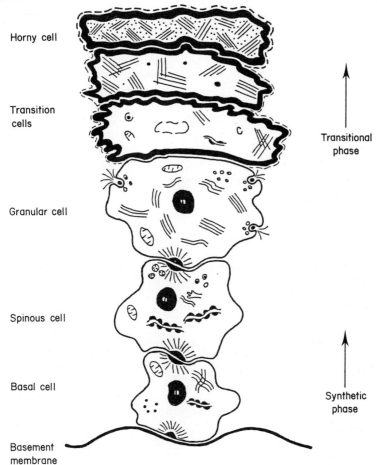

Horny cell

Transition
cells

Granular cell

Spinous cell

Basal cell

Basement
membrane

Transitional
phase

Synthetic
phase

Fig. 2–1   Diagram to show the cell types in human epidermis (not to scale). From the basement membrane moving 'outwards', the cell layers are (**1**) *stratum basale* or *stratum germinativum* (basal or germinative layer); (**2**) *stratum spinosum* (spinous layer or spinous cells); (**3**) *stratum granulosum* (granular layer); (**4**) *stratum lucidum* (transitional layer); (**5**) *stratum corneum* (horny layer of dead cells). Note that there are several layers (3–6) of each cell type except for the basal layer which is only 1–2 cells thick (see text). The thickness of the *stratum corneum* obviously depends partly on the rate of sloughing off of dead cells (see Fig. 2–2).

keratohyaline granules. The granular layer is most highly developed in the regions where abundant keratin is produced, namely the palmar and plantar regions. Electron microscopy shows the keratohyaline granules to be amorphous in structure, and it is now known that they contain the protein called filaggrin (see p. 11).

Above the granular layer, a single layer of cells lacking nuclei, the *stratum lucidum*, which appear to contain droplets of an oily substance, can sometimes be seen. This may be produced as a result of the disintegration of the lysosomes. The cells are probably representative of a step on the way to becoming the flat, anucleate, cornified dead cells which constitute the *stratum corneum*. This latter layer is rich in keratin, and varies in thickness depending on the region of the body, being thickest in palmar and plantar regions (Fig. 2–2). In these regions, which are subject to pressure, the layer of keratinized cells is dense and compact whereas over other regions it is more loose and flexible. In either case, however, the inert nature of the keratin renders the skin tough, pliable and relatively impermeable to substances passing in or out of the body.

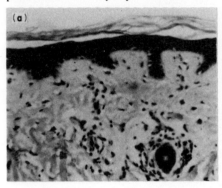
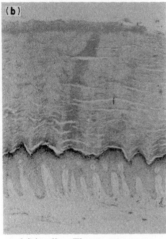

Fig. 2–2 Histological section of human (a) skin and (b) callus. The stratum corneum normally breaks away during the sectioning procedure. Note the greatly thickened stratum corneum in the callus.

It is worth pointing out at this stage that epidermis is peculiar in its behaviour by comparison with most other parts of the body. From the time the embryo has an epidermis until the individual is dead, the epidermis is continually producing new cells to be shed, eventually, from the surface. Few other tissues in the body behave like this and in some ways this behaviour is more reminiscent of that of cancerous cells. The growth of epidermal appendages such as nails and hair is also essentially continuous throughout life.

The major protein component of the dead cells of the stratum corneum is keratin and for this reason the transformation of cells into 'keratinocytes' is referred to as *keratinization*. This term encompasses the transition undergone by a living epidermal cell as it moves outwards to the exterior eventually forming a flattened dead cell of the stratum corneum.

2.2   The keratins

The fibrous protein keratin occurs in skin, hair, nails, claws, hoof and so on, but it should be made clear from the outset that the term 'keratin' is used to describe a large group of related proteins rather than a single substance. For example, the so-called 'hard' keratins that form hair and nail have quite different properties from the 'soft' keratins found in the cells of the stratum corneum. Hard keratins are rich in the sulphur-containing amino acid cysteine but soft keratins contain very little (Table 2–1). Nevertheless skin and hair keratins share some common features. It has been shown recently, for instance, that one of the skin keratins has an amino acid sequence that is 60% homologous with that of type I wool keratin and 38% homologous with that of type II keratin. Furthermore, it is now clear that the keratin tonofilaments form part of a much larger family of filamentous structures called *intermediate filaments*. The name 'intermediate' was given simply because such filaments have a diameter of between 8 and 11 nm and are therefore 'intermediate' in size between the other known filament-forming materials, namely actin (4 nm) and microtubules (25 nm). Examples of other intermediate filaments are *desmin* from muscle, which is thought to hold the myofibrils in place in the muscle bundles; *vimentin*, which occurs in many cells of mesenchymal origin and may be involved in mechanically supporting the cell nucleus or holding it in its place in the cell; and two classes of filament from nerve cells, *neurofilaments* and *glial filaments*. Now that some amino acid sequences are available it is possible to say that the filament-forming proteins are about 30% homologous with the skin keratins.

Table 2–1   Amino acid composition of human skin, nail and hair keratins expressed as residues per hundred residues. Tryptophan was not determined.

Amino acid	Skin prekeratin	Skin keratin	Nail*	Hair*
Cysteine (as cysteic acid)	0.4	0.5	7.4	7.6
Aspartic acid	9.2	10.3	8.9	9.3
Threonine	3.5	4.4	5.0	5.5
Serine	9.4	11.4	8.7	9.0
Glutamic acid	13.5	14.3	15.2	16.6
Proline	1.9	1.5	4.1	3.8
Glycine	18.5	22.8	6.6	5.2
Alanine	5.4	6.6	6.5	6.9
Valine	3.5	3.2	5.9	6.1
Methionine	3.1	0.7	0.8	0.4
Isoleucine	3.5	3.4	3.9	3.7
Leucine	8.9	9.7	9.9	10.2
Tyrosine	3.0	0.5	2.8	2.5
Phenylalanine	3.0	2.8	2.2	2.0
Lysine	4.8	5.0	4.5	3.5
Histidine	1.6	2.5	0.9	0.7
Arginine	6.7	4.5	6.7	7.2

*Taken from FRASER, R.D.B., MACRAE, T.P. and ROGERS, G.E. (1972). *Keratins – their composition, structure and biosynthesis*. Thomas, Springfield, IL, U.S.A.

Of the intermediate filament proteins, the keratins form by far the largest class. As would be expected of inert, insoluble proteins, quite harsh conditions are necessary to extract keratins from skin. Analysis of the keratins extracted from human epidermis using denaturing solvents (e.g. 8 M urea) to solubilize the polypeptides and reducing agents (e.g. 2-mercaptoethanol) to break disulphide bonds, reveals a family of polypeptides with molecular weights in the range 46 000–70 000 (Fig. 2–3). Somewhat milder conditions, for example low pH in the absence of reducing agents, also extract a number of polypeptides (Fig. 2–3). This latter set of polypeptides is referred to as 'prekeratin', the implication being that it is a precursor of the 'keratin' which is gradually formed as the cells move upwards from the basal layer, by a process involving the formation of disulphide cross-links as well as other changes.

The individual keratin filaments seem to have the in-built propensity to combine with one another to form filaments. Most combinations of two or

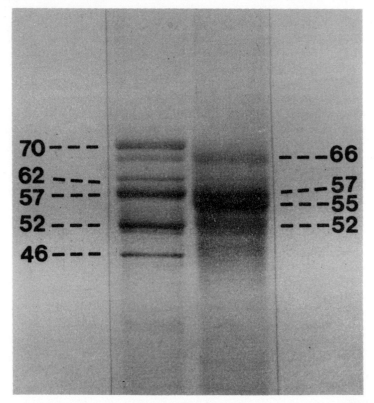

Fig. 2–3 Behaviour of human epidermal prekeratin (left) and keratin (right) in electrophoresis. The electrophoresis was performed in the presence of a detergent (SDS) so that the separation is according to relative molecular mass (M_r). The scales right and left give $M_r \times 10^{-3}$. It can be seen that there are at least 10 polypeptides in prekeratin and probably a similar number, but with a different M_r range, in keratin.

three purified keratin polypeptides seem to polymerize into filaments with the same general structure as native keratin, namely a characteristic rope-like morphology with a diameter of 8 nm and the characteristic X-ray diffraction pattern. It is believed that each polypeptide has two helical regions 100–120 amino acid residues in length, separated by a non-helical region, probably with non-helical regions at the ends. Earlier work had suggested that helical regions in different polypeptides came together to form a triple helix, but more recent work suggests that two polypeptides, not three, combine in this way. How such structures form the native filament remains to be seen. As already mentioned, electron microscopy shows that bundles of keratin filaments often terminate in membrane-bound desmosomes.

2.3 Keratinization

The cells of the basal layer are already synthesizing keratin, and in the spinous and granular cell layers the cells continue to be active biosynthetically. Later they are destined to lose most of their cellular organelles. In the spinous cell layer a characteristic organelle, typically 0.1–0.5 μm in diameter, surrounded by a 3 nm-thick membrane, may be observed. These granules have been variously called 'membrane-coating granules' 'Odland bodies', 'lamellated granules', 'keratinosomes' and 'cementsomes'. In the electron microscope they seem to have an ordered internal structure of parallel lamellae of alternating high and low densities. During the granular phase of keratinization they move towards the cell membrane and there seem to empty their contents into the intercellular spaces. The lamellar material is thought to form several layers of broad sheets which attach to the outer surfaces of the horny cells. This has the effect of filling all the gaps between cells so that the stratum corneum forms an effective barrier.

2.4 Keratohyaline granules

Another characteristic epidermal cell organelle is the keratohyaline granule which is observed in the granular layer. This stains blue with haematoxylin/ eosin and gives the granular layer its name and characteristic appearance. The granules are typically 100–200 μm in diameter and the number per cell varies from one region of the skin to another and even between cells in the same histological section. It is believed that the granules contain the precursor of a protein called *filaggrin*, which has also been called 'histidine-rich protein' and 'stratum corneum basic protein'. The name filaggrin is a contraction of 'filament-aggregating protein' and it is believed that it is concerned in some as yet unknown way with the organizing of large amounts of keratin filaments into an intracellular matrix.

2.5 Terminal differentiation

After leaving the granular cell layer the keratinocytes enter a transitional phase during which lysosomal enzymes become activated, resulting eventually in the breakdown of the nucleus and all the other cell organelles. During this phase the cells start to flatten and the cell membrane becomes strengthened by a process in which the cell envelope protein *involucrin* undergoes covalent crosslinking. Probably about half the 'life time' of an epidermal cell is spent undergoing differentiation. For the other half it exists as a dead keratinocyte which is eventually sloughed off from the surface as part of the wear and tear of the skin surface. The locking together of the flat cells along with the presence of lipid material (see below) makes a very effective barrier.

It is possible that there is a good deal of order in the way in which keratinocytes are formed and shed, although at present we know very little about the process. It has been shown that the stratum corneum of mouse ear comprises units in which groups of about six hexagonally-shaped cells are stacked one above the other into regular columns with minimal overlap between their counterparts in neighbouring columns. A somewhat similar arrangement can be seen in human epidermis, at least in some regions of the skin. In many cases the columns can be traced to the basal layer. The implication is that the pattern of *desquamation* is likely to be non-random and the migration from the basal layer is co-ordinated with the process of desquamation, at least under steady-state conditions.

2.6   The role of lipids

Lipid material probably makes up as much as 10% of the dry weight of the epidermis. (Dermis probably has much less, but it depends on the content of sebaceous glands and whether the layer of adipose tissue or 'hypodermis' is included.) The majority of the epidermal lipid is produced by the sebaceous glands which are epidermal in origin (p. 14) although they lie predominantly in the dermis.

The sebum probably has several functions. In humans it controls moisture loss from the epidermis and has been claimed to prevent fungal and bacterial infection. Certainly cornified epithelium, such as a cutting from a plantar callus, becomes hard and brittle if it is allowed to dry out. Treating cornified epithelium with organic solvents greatly reduces its water-holding capacity. Also it is a familiar experience that after washing the finger tips with solvents such as acetone, there is a tendency to drop things. This is a consequence of the fact that the layer of lipid on our finger tips enables us to perform delicate manipulations with a minimum of pressure. Another common experience is the drying out of the skin, and consequent chapping of the skin surface, under the lower relative humidities and temperatures of winter weather or in rapidly flowing air. In hairy mammals sebum is probably important in waterproofing the coat and in some mammals aggregations of holocrine gland units play an important part in scent production.

In areas of the skin where sebaceous glands are abundant, for example the scalp, forehead and upper back, as much as 90% of the surface lipid is of sebaceous origin and reflects the composition of sebum with reasonable accuracy. Analyses of such surface lipid may be compared with those of 'pure' sebum (Table 2–2). The presence of squalene is characteristic of sebum, and this compound is a known precursor of sterols such as cholesterol (Fig. 2–4).

Table 2–2 Percentage composition of sebum and epidermal lipid. (Taken from ROOK, A., WILKINSON, D.S. and EBLING, F.J.G. (1979). *Textbook of Dermatology*, third edition. Blackwell Scientific Publications, Oxford.)

Constituent	Sebum	Epidermal lipid
Glyceride, and free fatty acids	57.5	65
Wax esters	26.0	–
Squalene	12.0	–
Cholesterol	1.5	20
Cholesterol esters	3.0	15

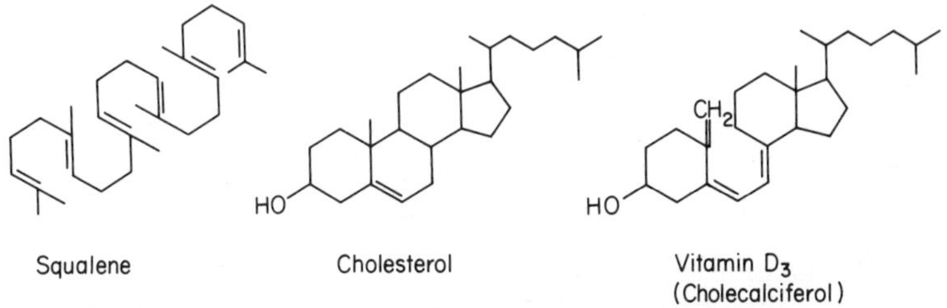

Squalene   Cholesterol   Vitamin D₃
                                        (Cholecalciferol)

Fig. 2–4 Some of the steroids and steroid-related compounds of human skin (see text): squalene, cholesterol and vitamin D_3. Cholesterol is normally formed in liver from its precursor squalene. Vitamin D_3 is formed in skin by the action of sunlight on $\Delta^{5,7}$-cholesterol.

However, it may be concluded that sebaceous glands do not to any great extent convert squalene to sterols. In contrast, in epidermis, squalene synthesized in the lower layers is almost totally converted to sterols, either to cholesterol or precursors of vitamin D.

Fatty acids, either free or esterified as glycerides, phospholipids, sterol esters or wax esters, constitute about 60% of both epidermal and sebum lipids. Many different types of fatty acid are found, but C16 and C18 fatty acids predominate. Although free fatty acids are abundant in surface lipids, they are present only in trace amounts in the contents of intact sebaceous cysts as well as in intact glands. This suggests that lipids synthesized in the sebaceous cells are modified during the intrafollicular transit of sebum. It is now well established that the free fatty acids present on the surface and in blackheads (see p. 58) are generated from serum triglycerides by the action of bacterial lipases.

There is no evidence that any components of sebum are directly derived from ingested fat. However, the composition and excretion rate *is* affected by hormones (see below). The amount of sebum secreted depends on a number of factors including the anatomical site. For example 5–10 μg sebum were recovered per square centimetre from the trunk and limbs of subjects who had washed 3 hours prior to extraction, compared with 150–300 μg cm^{-2} from the forehead.

2.7   The sebaceous gland

The sebaceous gland is holocrine and its secretion is produced by complete disintegration of the glandular cells. The development of the glands is very closely related to the differentiation of hair follicles and epidermis, and as already mentioned the glands are epidermal in origin (p. 12). In the human foetus, sebaceous glands are distinguishable by 13–15 weeks, and the central cells are seen to contain lipid droplets shortly after this. Thereafter the glands become multi-acinar and functional and indeed sebum is the first demonstrable glandular product of the human body. Interestingly, between birth and sexual maturity, the skin surface lipid undergoes distinct changes. Shortly after birth it is similar in composition to adult sebum, presumably because the glands have been activated by the maternal hormones. From the age of 2 until about 8 years the amounts of wax esters and squalene decline and cholesterol and its esters predominate. On the approach to puberty the levels of wax esters and squalene gradually rise until at about 15 years the composition comes to resemble that of the adult.

The sebaceous glands themselves consist of a series of lobes each with a duct lined by keratinizing squamous epithelium (Fig. 2–5). The ducts from the lobes converge and eventually the main duct, whose epithelium is continuous with

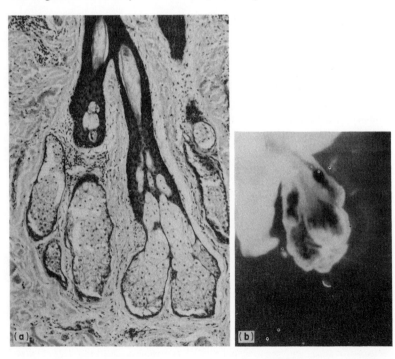

Fig. 2–5   (a) Histology of human sebaceous gland. The duct opens to the epidermis at the top of the picture. (b) A single gland that has been dissected from the dermis but remains attached to the underside of the epidermis.

the surface epidermis, carries sebum to the surface. Within a given unit the acini vary in extent of differentiation and maturity.

Sebaceous glands occur over much of the body but not normally on the palms and soles. On the scalp and forehead there may be 400–900 glands per cm^2 but elsewhere there tend to be less than 100 glands per cm^2. Most of the glands are associated with hair follicles to form the pilosebaceous unit (see below), but at a number of sites they open directly on to the skin surface not by way of a hair follicle. Such sites include the eyelids, the margin of upper lip and the areolae of the nipples.

Sebaceous gland activity is stimulated by androgens and it has been shown that administration of testosterone increases both the sebaceous gland size and the sebum output of pre-pubertal boys but not of adult males. Eunuchs secrete about half as much sebum as normal males. Adult women secrete, on the average, only a little less sebum than adult males. In contrast to this, oestrogens depress sebaceous activity, decreasing both the size of the glands and the rate of sebum output. The relationships between androgens and oestrogens and sebum output are poorly understood however. Some non-oestrogenic steroids (e.g. α-norprogesterone, cyproterone acetate) which antagonize the action of androgens at the target site can reduce sebaceous activity.

2.8   Hair

Hairs, as well as the sweat glands, are epidermal appendages that lie in the dermis. The hair is closely associated with sebaceous glands and will be dealt with here: sweat glands will be dealt with in Chapter 3 under the control of body temperature (p. 28).

Hairs grow out of tubular invaginations of the epidermal surface called follicles, and a follicle, together with its associated sebaceous gland is called a *pilosebaceous unit* (Fig. 2–6). The epidermis is continuous with the epithelium lining the pilosebaceous follicle. A small bundle of smooth muscle fibres, the *arrector pili*, joins the wall of the follicle to the epidermis. These muscles are supplied by adrenergic nerve fibres and are responsible for the erection of hairs during cold or emotional stress ('goose flesh'). The hair itself is almost wholly a dead structure, but at the base is a small growing area called the hair bulb. The shaft of the hair is keratinized and the junction between the living and dead regions is known as the keratinogenous zone.

All the follicles on the human scalp are established at birth and no new follicles form thereafter. The pattern and distribution, as well as the colour of hair are genetically determined. The hair bulb is situated in the upper part of the subcutaneous fat and is highly vascularized at the base. In people with dark hair the cells of the bulb contain large amounts of melanin (see p. 32) Interspersed among the cells of the bulb are dendritic melanocytes.

Cells are produced by the hair bulb and gradually elongate and undergo keratinization. The hair shaft is a keratinized structure composed of an outer cortex where the cells are cemented together very firmly, and an inner medulla where the cells are somewhat larger, more loosely connected and partially separated by air spaces. Hair growth is cyclical, and after a period of growth

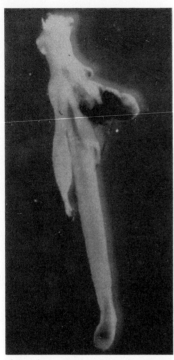

Fig. 2–6 A pilosebaceous unit, i.e. a hair sheath with its accompanying sebaceous gland. This was obtained by micro-dissection. The hair bulb is seen at the bottom of the picture. Approximate length, 4–5 mm.

there is a phase of regression. The lower part of the follicle degenerates, the hair loosens, and is eventually pushed out by the growth of a new hair. In young adult human scalp the growth phase is about three years in duration but this does not apply to the rest of the body where the growth phase is measured in months. In most hairy mammals there are synchronous cycles of follicular growth but in humans activity tends to be irregular and neighbouring follicles tend to be at different stages of their cycle.

The pattern and extent of hair growth is genetically determined in both males and females, but against this genetic background the hormones produce marked and characteristic effects. Before birth the human foetus has a coat of fine, soft, usually unpigmented hair known as *lanugo*. This is normally shed *in utero* at about the seventh or eighth month of gestation. Except on the head, the infant and child have 'vellus' hair, which is fine, short and non-pigmented, on all body surfaces save the palms and soles. At puberty, 'terminal' hair appears in the secondary sexual areas, starting in the pubic region (Fig. 2–7). This hair is pigmented and gradually becomes coarser and curly. The change to terminal hair in these sites is a programmed event in development but requires the presence of androgens, in both males and females, at puberty for its expression. Eunuchs and males castrated before puberty do not develop terminal hair unless they are given androgens. Despite this, however, there is no established quantitative relationship between plasma androgen levels and the extent of hair growth in men. Claims by bearded men that beards reflect masculinity are difficult to sustain.

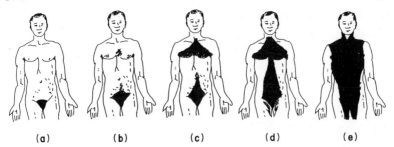

Fig. 2–7 The anatomical distribution of terminal body hair after puberty. (**a**) The typical female hair distribution pattern; (**b**) – (**e**) show the development and distribution of the male hair pattern. In the male pattern a beard is also typical, of course.

Axillary hair first appears about two years after the start of pubic hair growth, but thereafter males and females differ in that only males develop hair on the face, chest, back and limbs. The adult pattern (Fig. 2–7) is not fully achieved until the fourth decade when androgen levels are already lower than in early adulthood.

In the majority of men, at some time after puberty, certain follicles of the scalp may regress with age to produce only fine, short, vellus hair. This results in the so-called male-pattern baldness or 'androgenic alopecia'. This is the familiar 'receding at the temples' and development of a 'bald patch', with progressive extension with increasing age (Fig. 2–8). This type of baldness is inherited and occurs only in the presence of male hormone. It is prevented by castration before puberty although not substantially reversed by castration at maturity. It also occurs in chimpanzees, orangutans and other primates.

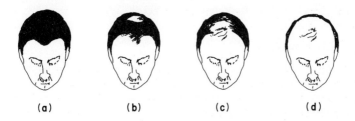

Fig. 2–8 Maturity onset alopecia (male baldness). Typical male pattern hair loss is shown diagrammatically in (**a**) – (**d**). The hair line on the temple recedes and there is development of a bald patch on the crown of the head.

The other phenomenon observed to occur with age is the greying of hair. The gradual loss of pigment in the hair shafts is associated with a progressive loss of tyrosinase activity by the melanocytes (see p. 32). In white hair melanocytes are practically absent. The age of onset of 'greying' is largely determined by inheritance but other factors may be involved such as severe emotional stress, cardiovascular disease, hyperthyroidism and some autoimmune diseases.

2.9   Nails

A nail is made of a more or less transparent plate of keratin surrounded by folds of skin called the nail folds. An area of modified epidermis, the nail bed, gives rise to the nail.

The nail itself consists of three parts: the root, the nail plate and the free edge (Fig. 2–9). The root is overlapped by the proximal nail fold, which is continuous with the lateral nail folds. The whitish area near to the root is called the *lunula* and overlying this is a thin cuticular fold, the *eponychium*. The lunula is usually completely visible on the thumbnail but tends to be covered on the fifth nail. Underneath the free margin of the nail is thickened epidermis, the *hyponychium*. The nail plate lies upon a vascularized nail bed. The horny layers of the nail bed and the nail plate are firmly attached and forward movement of the nail plate is accompanied by forward movement of keratinized cells on the nail bed. Human fingernails grow more quickly than toe nails, the times for replacement being about 6 months and 12–18 months respectively. Finger nails grow, on average, about 0.1 mm a day, growth being faster in summer than in winter.

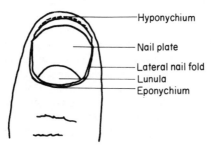

Fig. 2–9   Sketch to show the various parts of a nail.

2.10   Dermatoglyphics

Finger prints, the characteristic elevated ridge patterns on the finger tips of humans, are unique to the individual and serve as a means of identification (Fig. 2–10). Even identical twins have non-identical finger print patterns although the patterns do tend to be somewhat similar in this case. The term *dermatoglyphics* is applied both to the configurations of the ridges and to the study of 'finger prints'. The patterns appear in the foetus between weeks 13 and 19, the hand developing somewhat in advance of the foot.

In humans, the fingertip has one of three configurations, namely a whorl, a loop, or an arch. Arches may be simple or tented, loops are described as ulnar or radial according to which way they face, and whorls are divided into symmetrical, spiral or double loops. In Britain about 70% of people have loops, 25% have whorls and only 5% have arches.

It is also possible to distinguish six such configurational areas, each with its own discrete pattern, on the palms, but it is rare for a single hand to possess the entire complement.

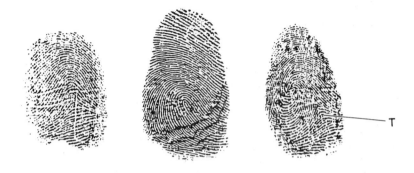

Fig. 2–10 Dermatoglyphs. Fingerprints have arches, loops and whorls.

The systematic classification of ridge patterns as a means of personal identification or for use in studies of inheritance, requires numerical procedures such as counting the number of ridges between specified points or measuring angles. Where different areas join are found deltas or tri-radii (T in Fig. 2–10): on a finger-tip a single tri-radius always accompanies a loop pattern and two accompany a whorl. When no tri-radii are present the pattern is referred to as an open field, or an arch. One method of counting and identification is to count the number of ridges crossed by a straight line drawn from the core of the pattern to the tri-radius.

A great deal of information has accumulated as a consequence of classification and forensic studies. Thus there are well-known statistical differences between left and right hands, between males and females, and between different races. For example, whorls are found more commonly in right than in left hands, and more commonly in Caucasoid males than Caucasoid females. Whorls are five times more abundant in Australian aboriginals than in some groups of Africans. Distortions of the dermatoglyphic pattern occur in a number of chromosomal aberrations. Sometimes dermatoglyphic features can indicate an increased liability to develop a particular medical condition and may be a useful aid to diagnosis. In the well-known Down's Syndrome (mongolism or G trisomy) about a third of patients have ten ulnar loops whereas only about 4% of normal individuals have this arrangement. In Klinefelter's syndrome (males have 47 chromosomes with sex chromosome constitution XXY, psychologically male but sterile) the total ridge count is reduced, and arch patterns are increased. In contrast, in females with Turner's Syndrome (45 chromosomes, XO, i.e. lacking Y sex chromosome, high neonatal mortality, short stature, high incidence of congenital defects) the total ridge count tends to be much increased. Deficient ridge formation is rarely seen in normal individuals (<1%) but is reported to occur in nearly 20% of cases of schizophrenia. In psoriasis (see p. 60) there is an increase in the incidence of whorls in the fourth digit, particularly in the right hand. Fingerprints are an example of polygenic inheritance, i.e. many genes control a single character.

3 The Dermis

3.1 Introduction

The dermis forms the bulk of the skin. It is a tough, resilient tissue that cushions underlying organs against mechanical injury and provides nutriment for the epidermis and cutaneous appendages (see Fig. 1–1). The main structural feature of the dermis is a network of mechanically strong fibres, mostly *collagen*, but with some *elastin*, embedded in a matrix of amorphous ground substance. The fibres (collagen, elastin) are protein and the ground substance is polysaccharide (see below). In contrast to the epidermis which is almost entirely cellular, the dermis contains few cells. Most of these are fibroblasts which are responsible for secreting the dermal constituents, but mast cells (p. 46), macrophages and lymphocytes, and melanocytes (p. 32) are also present. The dermis also has vascular beds at various levels, lymphatics, nerves and various types of nerve ending.

3.2 The function of the dermis

The main function of the dermis is mechanical. When normal skin is stretched, the irregular, three-dimensional network of collagen fibres gradually becomes re-orientated into an arrangement of more parallel bundles. There is a complex interrelationship between the biomechanical properties of skin, however, which give it its capacity to adapt to local or general changes in size and contour, to allow for movement of head and limbs, and, especially in humans, to allow for a very wide range of facial expressions. The biomechanical properties result from the interplay of three factors:

(1) *tension*, or resistance to deforming forces, which is provided by the elastic fibres;

(2) *elasticity*, or the ability to resume its original shape after the deforming forces have ceased to act; and

(3) *tensile strength*, which depends mainly on the collagen fibres, and is the degree to which elongation can take place before tearing occurs.

One or all of these properties may be absent as a result of congenital disease (see p. 62) or may be modified by disease or by ageing.

The collagen fibres, which can form up to 30% by volume of the dermis, have a high tensile strength but very little elasticity. It is said that collagen fibrils can support at least 10 000 times their own weight. The return to normal after stretching depends mainly on the elastin fibres which constitute only about 1% of the volume of the dermis. Over-extension can occur, for example in pregnancy or rapidly developing obesity, leading to rupture of the elastic fibres, allowing the collagen to become over-stretched. This results in characteristic linear scars within the dermis called *striae*.

In addition to this mechanical role, the dermis also acts as a supporting tissue. The dermis itself arises from the embryological mesoderm. However during foetal life the various epidermal appendages (sweat glands, apocrine glands, sebaceous glands, hair and nails) arise from the undersurface of the developing epidermis. In the human foetus, small buds of cells or primary epithelial germs appear at about the third month. From these the hair matrix, the sebaceous glands and the apocrine glands develop. Sweat buds appear on the palms and soles during the fourth month of embryonic life; those of the axillae and the rest of the body surface develop later.

In vertical section the boundary between dermis and epidermis is wavy. The upward projections of dermis are called *dermal papillae* (Fig. 3–1), interdigitating with downward projections of epidermis called *rete ridges*. The basement membrane which lies at the junction of dermis and epidermis is largely formed by the basal cells, and includes amongst its components type IV, or basal membrane type collagen, which has special and distinct properties compared with dermal or other types of collagen (see Table 3–1).

In addition to its mechanical and supporting roles the dermis exerts an inductive influence during development on the structure and differentiation of the epidermis. It seems likely that this influence continues into adult life as changes in the dermis often precede the development of cancers of the epidermis (see p. 65).

3.3   Collagen

Most cells in a multicellular organism are in contact with an extracellular meshwork of interacting macromolecules which constitute the *extracellular matrix* and this is particularly true of dermis. The protein and polysaccharide molecules forming this matrix are secreted locally and assemble into an organized meshwork which, until recently, was thought to serve mainly as an inert scaffolding. However, it is now clear that it has a much more complex and active role in regulating the behaviour of the cells in contact with it. We know something of the chemical and physical properties of the major types of molecules that constitute the extracellular matrix, but much remains to be discovered.

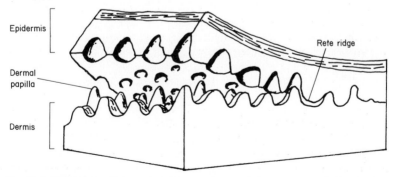

Fig. 3–1 Schematic diagram to show dermal papillae at the interface between epidermis and dermis.

The molecules of the extracellular matrix are secreted by the fibroblasts which are widely distributed in the matrix. The long, strong collagen fibres help to strengthen and organize the matrix, the elastin fibres provide elasticity, while the aqueous phase of polysaccharide gel permits the diffusion of nutrients, metabolites and hormones between the blood and tissue cells.

'Collagen' comprises a group of proteins which are in fact the most abundant proteins of mammals, constituting about 25% of the body weight. They have highly characteristic amino acid compositions and sequences and their major structural feature is the ability to form a stiff, triple-stranded helical structure about 300 nm long and 1.5 nm in diameter. The three collagen polypeptides that are wound together in the triple helix are called α-chains, and so far seven genetically-distinct α-chains have been characterized (Table 3–1). Type I collagen is the most predominant (about 90%) in vertebrates, including vertebrate dermis, but some type III collagen is also present. As mentioned above, type IV collagen is characteristic of basement membranes.

Collagen polypeptides are synthesized on membrane-bound ribosomes as precursors which are larger than the final polypeptides. These are called pro-collagen polypeptides and are characterized by having 'extension peptides' at both ends. These polypeptides pass into the endoplasmic reticulum space and there each pro-collagen polypeptide combines with two others to form a hydrogen-bonded, triple-stranded helix. It seems likely that the extension peptides have an important role to play in guiding proper triple helix formation. Later they are removed by specific enzymes called pro-collagen peptidases, and the remaining triple helical sections come together in the extracellular space to form much larger collagen fibrils. However, this is not true of type IV, or basement membrane collagen, which seems to retain its extension peptides. In the electron microscope isolated collagen fibrils exhibit cross-striations every 67 nm and this pattern is believed to reflect the packaging

Table 3–1 Types of collagen.

Type	Structure of triple helix*	Distinctive features	Distribution
I	$[1(I)]_2\,2(I)$	Low carbohydrate	Skin, tendon, bone, cornea (over 90% of collagen)
II	$[1(II)]_3$	High carbohydrate	Cartilage
III	$[1(III)]_3$	High hydroxyproline, low carbohydrate	Skin, blood vessels
IV	$[1(IV)]_3$	High carbohydrate, retains extension peptides	Basal lamina
V	$[1(V)]_2\,2(V)$	High carbohydrate	Widespread in small amounts

* Seven different types of polypeptide are known at present, designated 1(I) to 1(V), 2(I) and 2(V). These types also have a high content of the modified amino acid hydroxy-lysine: type IV collagen is especially rich in this amino acid.

arrangement of the individual collagen molecules in the fibril (Fig. 3–2). Individual collagen molecules are displaced longitudinally by approximately one quarter of their length (i.e. 67 nm).

Collagen α-chains have an unusual amino acid composition being very rich in glycine and proline. These are extremely important in triple helix formation and indeed it is only because glycine effectively has no side-chain R-group that it is small enough to occupy the crowded interior of the triple helix. Practically every third residue along the polypeptide is glycyl.

Many of the prolines (and some lysines) are subsequently hydroxylated, and probably these hydroxyl groups participate in interchain hydrogen bonds that help to stabilize the triple helix. In the human disease, scurvy, a dietary deficiency of vitamin C (ascorbic acid) leads to the inability to hydroxylate proline residues properly and consequently the collagen formed is weaker. In scurvy sufferers the skin and blood vessels are extremely fragile and bleeding into the tissues is a common feature.

It is not known what controls the way in which the collagen fibrils are laid down in the extracellular matrix. For example in mammalian skin the collagen fibrils appear to be dispersed randomly in the ground substance whereas in

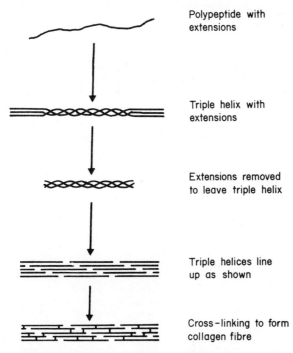

Polypeptide with extensions

Triple helix with extensions

Extensions removed to leave triple helix

Triple helices line up as shown

Cross–linking to form collagen fibre

Fig. 3–2 Sketch to show the formation of mature collagen. Polypeptides synthesized on the ribosomes are hydroxylated and glycosylated and then assemble to form a triple helix (of pro-collagen). After secretion from the cell into the extracellular matrix, the pro-collagen peptides are cleaved and the collagen triple helices form fibrils. Subsequently cross-links are formed.

tendons, the fibrils are organized into parallel bundles for maximum strength along the major axis of stress.

After the collagen fibrils have formed in the extracellular space, they are considerably strengthened by the formation of covalent cross-links within and between the constituent collagen molecules. These links are mostly between lysine residues. However, in addition, some of the lysine residues in the collagen polypeptides have sugar residues attached to them. This modification seems to take place before the molecules leave the cells. The amount of carbohydrate added varies greatly with the type of collagen. For example, skin collagens contain relatively low amounts of carbohydrates whereas cartilage collagen is rich in carbohydrate. The function of this carbohydrate component is not known although it is possible that it has a role in the interaction with the ground substance in which the collagen fibrils are embedded.

3.4   Elastin

Elastin is a protein of relative molecular mass about 70 000. Like collagen it is unusually rich in proline and glycine residues but little hydroxyproline is present. Elastin molecules secreted into the extracellular space form filaments and sheets in which the molecules are extensively cross-linked to form a

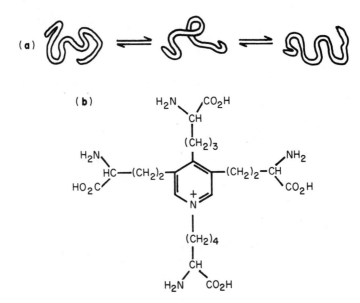

Fig. 3–3 Elastin. The polypeptide chain of elastin (**a**) does not have a unique conformation but remains as a partially-folded 'random coil' that can adopt a number of conformations. In addition the molecules are cross-linked. Four lysin residues in different polypeptides come together and the compound desmosine (**b**) is formed, covalently linking the chains. The cross-linked, random coil structure give the material a highly elastic nature.

network. Lysine-rich regions of the polypeptides engage in the formation of covalent cross-links: four lysyl residues come together and are converted enzymically to desmosine. The cross-linked, random-coil structure so formed allows the material to stretch and recoil like rubber (Fig. 3–3). The interweaving of long but inelastic collagen fibrils sets a limit to the extent of stretching and hence prevents the tissue from tearing.

3.5   The ground substance

The ground substance in which collagen and elastin are embedded is made of a carbohydrate material now known as *glycosaminoglycan* but previously called muco-polysaccharide. This term encompasses a whole group of compounds, whose structures are closely similar. The basic feature of all the molecules is that they are long, unbranched polysaccharides composed of a repeating disaccharide unit (Table 3–2). One of the two monosaccharides in the disaccharide unit is always an amino sugar (e.g. N-acetylglucosamine or N-acetylgalactosamine). Sulphate groups are also present (except in hyaluronic acid, see Table 3–2) on the monosaccharides. The consequence of the presence of these as well as carboxylic acid grouping is that the molecules have a high negative charge and are very hydrophilic. With the exception of hyaluronic acid, all of these glycosaminoglycans are covalently linked to protein molecules to form *proteoglycans* which contain 90–95% carbohydrate

Table 3–2   The features of the glycosaminoglycans found in skin.

Glycosaminoglycan	M_r	Repeating disaccharide unit* $- (A - B)_n -$		Sulphates per disaccharide unit
Hyaluronic acid	Up to 8×10^6	D-glucuronic acid	N-acetyl-glucosamine	0
Chondroitin sulphate	5000–50 000	D-glucuronic acid	N-acetyl-galactosamine	0.2–2.0
Dermatan sulphate	15 000–40 000	L-iduronic acid	N-acetyl-galactosamine	1.0–2.0
Heparin	6000–25 000	L-iduronic acid	N-acetyl-glucosamine	2.0–3.0

* Example: dermatan sulphate

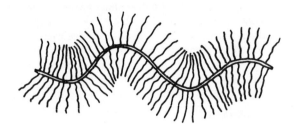

Fig. 3–4 Proteoglycans have a 'bottle-brush' type of structure with a polypeptide core and glycosaminoglycan 'bristles'. The whole molecule is 300 nm long. The core polypeptide (about 1800 amino acids) has a glycosaminoglycan every twelfth amino acid residue (serine). The sugar chains are relatively rigid, and, being hydrophilic and charged, attract water molecules. These will be squeezed out when pressure is applied but will rush back when it is released.

by weight. A typical proteoglycan might consist of a core peptide of about 1900 amino acids with, linked to it via serine residues, about 160 chondroitin sulphate (and perhaps other) polysaccharide glycosaminoglycan units in a 'bottle-brush' sort of formation (Fig. 3–4). Such molecules tend to adopt highly extended random-coil configurations which occupy a high volume for their mass. Since they are very hydrophilic they attract large amounts of water to form a hydrated gel. This tendency is enhanced by the presence of the negatively-charged groups which tend to attract osmotically active cations. The effect of applying pressure to such a gel is temporarily to squeeze out the water molecules, which rush back when the pressure is removed. Thus the gel has resilience and because of its porous and highly hydrated structure water-soluble molecules may easily and rapidly diffuse through the extracellular space.

Hyaluronic acid is somewhat different in lacking sulphate, having very long chains, and in not being joined to a protein core. It is produced in large amounts in tissues through which cells are migrating during development or wound healing, and it is possible that hyaluronic acid attracts water and swells the matrix, thus facilitating cell migration.

3.6 Dermal cells

As mentioned earlier, the dermis, in comparison with the epidermis is comparatively poor in cells, being composed mainly of connective tissue. The most abundant cell type is the *fibroblast*. This has a prominent, more or less round nucleus and the cell tends to be drawn out into a number of projections. In tissue culture, fibroblasts can be seen to move about. The cells form thin, sheet-like extensions from their leading edges, some of which form attachments to the substratum. Many, however, are carried back in a sweeping wave-like motion, called 'ruffling', on the upper surface of the cell. In the electron microscope the cytoplasm is observed to contain well-developed rough endoplasmic reticulum, pinocytotic vesicles, lysosomes and other granules. In tissues that are actively growing, for example around a healing wound, the fibroblasts are highly active.

There is no doubt that the fibroblasts produce collagen (or rather pro-collagen) but the status of these cells in relation to the production of elastin is less clear and the same applies to the production of ground substance. There is controversy, some authorities maintaining that fibroblasts produce all the materials of the extracellular matrix, while others hold that special cells, ('elastoblasts') produce elastin and yet others that the mast cells produce the glycosaminoglycans.

Mast cells are mentioned later (p. 46): here we need only note that they are relatively common in connective tissue, including dermis, along with macrophages. Macrophages, also called wandering histiocytes or phagocytic cells, originate from blood stem cells. In some connective tissue they are almost as abundant as fibroblasts from which they may be distinguished by having an indented, bean-shaped nucleus. Injection of a dye such as colloidal trypan blue into dermis shows an essential difference beween fibroblasts and macrophages: only the macrophages accumulate particles of the dye. This demonstrates the role of macrophages as scavengers of foreign particles, fragments of cells or extracellular material. Another difference is found in their distribution. Fibroblasts tend to occur near collagen fibres whereas macrophages tend to congregate in the region of blood vessels.

3.7   Changes with ageing

Collagen changes both qualitatively and quantitatively throughout life. In humans concentration of insoluble, deposited collagen increases from infant to adult, but from early adulthood onwards there is a gradual decrease in the absolute amount of collagen per unit area of skin. This is correlated with the characteristic change in appearance during ageing which occurs more rapidly in women than in men. Obviously, any change in the components of the dermis with age will affect the gross appearance of the skin. In addition to thickening of the epidermis, dependent to a great extent on the degree of exposure to sunlight (see p. 37), there will be changes in skin tone and elasticity.

3.8   Dermal appendages

The epidermis is an epithelium derived from ectoderm and the dermis is derived from mesoderm. As already mentioned keratinized appendages such as hairs, feathers and scales, as well as the various types of gland, form from epidermis. The structure and function of the sebaceous gland and of hair has already been described (p. 14), and it is well established that the dermis controls the character of the appendages as well as their physical arrangement. This can be seen especially vividly in the chick embryo. If embryonic leg epidermis, which would normally form scales, is removed and transplated over embryonic back dermis, which normally underlies feathers, then feathers, rather than scales, develop from leg epidermis. Similar experiments have been performed with mammalian epidermis taken from hairy and non-hairy regions.

3.9   Blood supply and temperature control

The cutaneous blood supply brings nourishment to the skin but it also has an important role in the regulation of body temperature. The skin itself is relatively modest in its requirements for oxygen but despite this it has a very abundant blood supply. An arterial twig penetrates the subcutaneous fat and forms a plexus just below the dermis. Another plexus is formed just below the papillary layer of the dermis (see Fig. 1–1) and loops extend upwards from this to individual dermal papillae, supplying the glands and hair roots. The epidermis is of course avascular, receiving its supply of nourishment from the vessels in the tips of the papillae, and presumably obtaining at least some of its oxygen by inward diffusion from the surface. Each individual arterial twig supplies a volume shaped like an inverted cone with the base towards the epidermis. This can be observed on cold hands and feet as a reticulate pattern. There is also a rich supply of lymphatic vessels in the dermis. These start at the tips of the papillae and pass between connective tissue fibres to join up, eventually, with the larger blood vessels. Blood collects into venous plexuses below the arterial plexuses, but arteriovenous shunts known as *glomus bodies* situated in various regions of the skin, allow the capillary circulation to be short-circuited. By shunting the blood in this way less heat may be lost, and *vice versa*. Glomus bodies are especially abundant in the pads of fingers and toes, the palms and soles, the ears and the central part of the face.

On exposure to heat the peripheral regions of the body become perfused by warm blood flowing through a widely dilated peripheral network. In contrast, upon exposure to cold, the rate of blood flow through the skin falls. If cold exposure is prolonged then heat production is increased either by voluntary movement or by shivering. These changes in body temperature are sensed by nerve endings with the hypothalamus acting as a co-ordinating centre.

3.10   Sweat glands

In conditions of great heat stress the sweat glands pour large quantities of fluid on to the body surface. In a relatively dry atmosphere the evaporation of this sweat can maintain a relatively satisfactory skin and body temperature.

Sweat glands are found over the whole surface of the skin but are particularly abundant on the palms and soles. In the human there are between two and five million sweat glands and there is some evidence of racial differences. The Japanese, for example, seem to have more sweat glands on the extremities than on the trunk, the distribution in Europeans being the opposite way round.

A sweat gland is a simple tubular gland extending from the epidermis, from which it is derived, to the mid-dermis where it becomes coiled upon itself. Two types of secreting epithelial cells can be recognized in the body of the gland, one small with a basophilic cytoplasm, the other larger with an acidophilic cytoplasm. The functional significance of these is not known. Sweat glands are described as *merocrine* organs because, unlike the holocrine sebaceous glands (p. 14), the cells are not destroyed in the process of secretion of sweat. Merocrine glands are further subdivided into apocrine and eccrine – apocrine glands secrete by a 'decapitation' of the apical cytoplasm of the epithelial cells, whereas no breakdown of any cellular material occurs at all in eccrine glands. However there is some controversy about this classification as applied to the sweat glands and some authorities have recommended distinguishing between those tubular glands which, like the sebaceous gland, normally develop from the external root sheath of the hair follicle and remain attached to it ('epitrichial'), and those which are independent ('atrichial'). Often epitrichial glands are referred to as apocrine glands. In humans eccrine (atrichial) glands are found over the whole skin surface but not on the mucous membranes. The numbers range from about 100 cm^{-2} on thigh to over 600 cm^{-2} on the soles of the feet.

In contrast the apocrine (epitrichial) glands, which are present throughout the skin surface in the embryo, mostly disappear subsequently so that in the adult they are found in the axillae, perianal region and the areoles of the breasts. These tend to be considerably larger than eccrine glands and are situated in the subcutaneous tissue. They secrete very small quantities of an oily fluid which is said to be odourless upon reaching the surface but thereafter develops a characteristic odour as a result of bacterial decomposition. These glands play no part in thermoregulation but may be relics of the glands found in many mammals which produce odours responsible for territory marking, species recognition or act as sex attractants.

Sweat, from the eccrine glands, is a clear, watery fluid of slightly acid pH, which contains salt, glucose and some nitrogenous substances (Table 3–3). However, the composition of sweat varies greatly from person to person, from time to time and from site to site as well as in health and disease. It is basically similar to a protein-free filtrate of the plasma from which it is derived, but the

Table 3–3 Composition of sweat. The latent heat of evaporation of 1 litre of sweat removes 2400 kJ from the body. At a maximal rate of about one litre an hour, the profusely sweating body can dispose of 25 kJ of heat per minute under suitable conditions, i.e. low relative humidity. The composition of plasma is shown for comparison.

	Composition of sweat (meq l^{-1})	Composition of plasma (meq l^{-1})
Sodium	20–70	137–148
Potassium	5–15	3.9–5.0
Chloride	20–76	100–106
Lactate	10–30	68–112
Urea	4–20 (mmol l^{-1})	2.7–5.8 (mmol l^{-1})
Glucose	0–3 (mg 100 ml^{-1})	68–96 (mg 100 ml^{-1})
Total osmolarity	100–200 m.osmol l^{-1} (hypotonic)	290 m.osmol l^{-1}
pH	4.0–6.5	7.4

sweat duct modifies its composition as it passes through. When sweat is flowing rapidly there will be little opportunity for modification.

Sweat glands are abundantly supplied with blood vessels which form a network around the secreting coils. These vessels are derived from a single arterial twig and are profusely supplied with cholinergic fibres from the sympathetic nervous system. Thermal sweating is controlled by the heat-regulating centre in the hypothalamus, which is activated by changes in blood temperature, and by afferent stimuli from the skin. Mental and emotional activity produce some increase in sweating especially on the palms and soles. Possibly this increases the grip at times of activity, but the nerve centres and pathways controlling mental sweating are not properly understood.

'Gustatory sweating' ('hyperhidrosis') is caused by eating spicy foods, and sweat secretion is also stimulated by nausea, fever, alcohol, and by certain drugs such as aspirin. In contrast sweat secretion is inhibited by atropine. Many compounds have been tried as 'anti-perspirants', including formaldehyde and glutaraldehyde. Most of the preparations on the market at the present time contain aluminium salts. Aluminium chloride hexahydrate, for example, is widely used in such preparations. It has a proven efficacy and its mechanism of action is partly understood. Aluminium (and other metabolic compounds with anti-perspirant properties) seem to cause mechanical obstruction of the eccrine sweat duct. Probably the metal ions form complexes with muco-polysaccharides that then precipitate. They may also damage the luminal epithelial cells thus generating an obstructive conglomerate. The secretory portion of the gland is not affected and remains active.

'Prickly heat' (milaria), a condition often experienced in hot weather, is produced in certain areas of the body as a consequence of obstruction of the sweat ducts followed by leakage of sweat into the surrounding area so that small, thin-walled vesicles form around the duct of the sweat gland. Milaria can occur, under heat stress, in sites rendered 'anhidrotic' by application of aluminium chloride.

3.11 Innervation

The skin is the major interface of the body with the environment and, not surprisingly, the skin is richly supplied with nerve endings which are constantly transmitting information about the environment to the brain. 'Cutaneous sensibility' includes the ability to detect changes in temperature, a sense of touch and pressure, sensitivity to vibrations, and ultimately the ability to experience pain. Many of the sensory neurones terminate in specialized receptors (see below) but many end in unmyelinated free-nerve endings. In the skin these latter tend to form plexuses from which fine branches penetrate between the cells. They probably have to do with the sense of touch and of pain.

At least five types of receptors are known which are responsible for skin sensibility (Fig. 3–5). *Meissner's corpuscles*, for example, are very abundant in the palmar skin of the fingertips and lie in rows on the dermal papillae (see Fig. 3–1). They contain horizontally stacked, flattened laminar cells and enable us to make discriminatory judgements by touch. They are probably responsible for our ability to recognize exactly what point on the body is touched and to recognize the texture of the objects touched. *Merkel's corpuscles*, which are disc shaped axon terminals applied to certain spherical 'clear' cells in the epidermis, probably send a steady signal that allows the perception of continuous touch of objects against the skin.

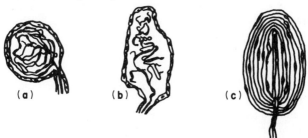

Fig. 3–5   Sketch to show the characteristic shapes of nerve receptors found in skin. (**a**) Krause end-bulbs are probably temperature sensitive; (**b**) Meissner's corpuscles are probably sensitive to superficial touch; and (**c**) Pacinian corpuscles are probably sensitive to pressure.

Ramifications of free nerve endings enclosed in capsules of connective tissue form *Krause end bulbs* (bulbous in shape) or *Ruffini terminals* (flattened in shape), and these, together with *Pacinian corpuscles* (see below), are present in the dermis but not epidermis, and respond to various cutaneous stimuli. It has proved difficult to identify particular responses with specific endings. Although we know that Meissner's corpuscles respond to light touch and that Pacinian corpuscles respond to pressure, there does not seem to be a tidy separation of sensory fibres into those signalling touch, temperature or damage to tissue.

Pacinian corpuscles are abundant in dermis and subcutaneous tissue but also occur in deep structures including nervous membranes, joints, tendons and so on. They seem to be involved in sensing vibration and in the perception of pressure. The response of these receptors is highly complicated and is poorly understood at present. Stimulation of a sensory ending gives rise to a receptor potential which appears at the specialized end of an afferent nerve fibre. This receptor potential is not an all-or-none phenomenon but varies in electrical size and time course. In some, but not all cases, the firing frequency of the nerve rapidly falls away, a process known as adaptation. For example, the Pacinian corpuscle and the receptors at hair bases adapt extremely rapidly. These obviously can only transmit information about *changes*. Other receptors, such as the Ruffini endings and Merkel's discs, adapt very poorly and continue to transmit information for many hours. This continued transmission gives the brain information on the state of a particular part of the body and its relationship to the surroundings. These types of receptor are known as *tonic* receptors while those giving information about changes are known as *rate receptors* or *phasic receptors*.

4 Melanogenesis

4.1 Introduction

The colour of skin and of hair arises as a result of a number of factors, some of which are non-pigmentous such as optical diffraction, light scattering and interference, and some of which result because of the presence of pigments. In skin, haemoglobin (in the blood vessels), and the yellow carotenoid pigments derived from plants (which accumulate in the lipid), make a contribution, but the fundamental colouring pigments are the red-to-black melanins. Indeed the melanins are amongst the most widespread natural pigments, being found in practically all living organisms including bacteria. They are responsible, for example, for the colours of bird feathers and of amphibian and reptilian skins.

Although the chemical structures of the melanins are highly complex and are only partially elucidated, there is now little doubt that all are derived ultimately from the amino acid, tyrosine, in a process requiring the participation of the enzyme *tyrosinase*. The biological functions of the melanins include protection of the underlying tissues against the deleterious effects of ultraviolet radiation in sunlight, heat control, and adaptive colouration. In mammalian, including human, skin, special cells called melanocytes, mesodermal in embryonic origin, are the basic units responsible for skin and hair pigmentation.

4.2 Melanocytes

The human body contains about two billion melanocytes, distributed throughout the body, mostly in the superficial epidermis, hair follicles and eye, but with lesser numbers elsewhere including some neural tissues that are hardly likely ever to be exposed to ultraviolet radiation. In skin there are on average about 1500 melanocytes per mm^2 but the figure varies depending upon the anatomical site. Perhaps surprisingly there are no significant racial differences: differences in skin colour are due to differences in packaging, distribution and degradation of the pigment organelles or melanosomes (see below).

The majority of the melanocytes in skin are found within the basal layer of epidermal cells (Fig. 4–1) and are roughly triangular cells with numerous fine, branching processes which can transfer melanin granules to the surrounding keratinocytes. A melanocyte together with its surrounding group of keratinocytes is sometimes referred to as an 'epidermal melanin unit'. Special staining procedures reveal melanocytes in histological sections in the light microscope, and in the electron microscope the presence of abundant rough endoplasmic reticulum indicates an actively secreting cell type.

Melanin is synthesized from tyrosine in melanocytes in numerous specialized cytoplasmic organelles called melanosomes. The enzyme tyrosinase is synthesized in the endoplasmic reticulum and transported to the Golgi region

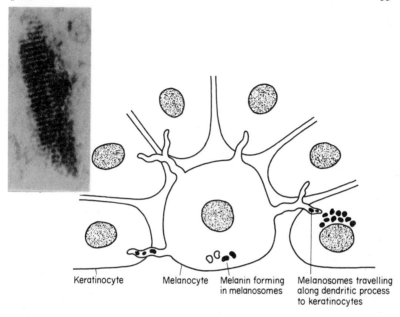

Fig. 4–1 Sketch to show a melanocyte in the basal layer of the epidermis, with its dendritic processes via which melanosomes pass to the keratinocytes. **Inset**: electron micrograph of a single melanosome.

where it is segregated into membrane-bound vesicles. These enlarge, become oval and acquire a characteristic internal structure, appearing in the electron microscope as a string of beads. This structure is referred to as a premelanosome and synthesis of melanin now commences. The granule gradually becomes more and more opaque as more melanin is laid down, and no internal structure can now be seen. The mature melanosome is a dense, homogeneous oval body, still inside the Golgi membrane, but is by now essentially devoid of tyrosinase.

At this stage the melanosomes can pass along the dendritic process of the melanocyte, to be 'injected' into the cytoplasm of the neighbouring basal layer keratinocytes. There is some evidence that transfer of melanin granules to keratinocytes involves active 'phagocytosis' of the melanin granule-filled tips of the dendritic processes of the melanocytes. In other words the basal cell is not simply a passive recipient and appears to take an active part in the process of transfer.

Inside the keratinocytes the granules tend to cluster as a protective cap over the cell nucleus. The keratinocytes eventually migrate upwards towards the stratum corneum and the melanosomes disintegrate or are eventually shed in the squames from the surface of the horny layer. Black skin contains no more melanocytes than white skin, but the melanosomes produced are larger and are dispersed rather than being in clumps. They may also be more resistant to degradation.

4.3   Melanogenesis

Although the chemical structure of the melanin pigments are by no means fully elucidated, enough is known for us to be able to speculate on the types of structure that may be found. Most of the information has come from the study of melanin formation, or 'melanogenesis', which has as its unifying feature the action of the ubiquitous tyrosinase enzyme. The key step in the process may be described in chemical terms as the enzymic conversion of a phenol (tyrosine) to the corresponding *ortho*quinone which then spontaneously undergoes extensive polymerization.

Orthoquinones are amongst the most chemically reactive of all organic compounds: the reactions they undergo include not only polymerization but also reductions, and reductive additions.

There are, broadly speaking, two types of melanin, the black-to-brown *eumelanins*, and the yellow-to-reddish brown *phaeomelanins*. These classifications were originally based on the distinction of the colours of hair by the naked eye, for example the 'red' of red hair being due to phaeomelanin. However it is now clear that there is a close relationship between the two pigment types and their biosynthetic origin, the main difference being that the sulphur-containing amino acid, cysteine, is involved in the production of phaeomelanins but not the eumelanins. It seems highly likely that the two 'pathways' of melanin biosynthesis overlap to some extent; and certainly it can be envisaged that, in the polymerization process, 'bystanding' molecules could easily become incorporated into the polymer.

In addition to the eumelanins and the phaeomelanins, there are low molecular weight melanoid pigments, *trichochromes*, which have a variety of colours from yellow to violet. An example of one such compound (which is yellow) is trichochrome C.

Several such pigments are known, each having a different colour, in hair and feathers. By comparison with the structures of phaeomelanins (see below) it is likely that these pigments have very similar biogenetic origins to the phaeomelanins.

Whatever the nature of the final pigment material that is finally formed, the initial step in melanin biogenesis is always the tyrosinase reaction. Tyrosinase is a copper-containing oxidase enzyme, and by its action the amino acid tyrosine is converted, in an oxidative step, to the compound called 'DOPA', which is a mnemonic for dihydroxyphenylalanine. In a second step also catalysed by tyrosinase this compound is converted into the orthoquinone, dopaquinone.

Tyrosine   DOPA   Dopaquinone

The scheme in Fig. 4–2 shows the two major routes by which eumelanins or phaeomelanins may be formed, largely spontaneously, and depending on whether or not cysteine becomes incorporated. Thus the fate of the dopaquinone, once formed, presumably depends to a considerable extent on the biochemical environment within the melanocyte, and not on enzymes. However, as is well known, there is also genetic control of the process, red-hair due to phaeomelanin, for example, being hereditary. Little is known about how this genetic control is achieved.

The type of granule formed with the different pigments, is in itself different, and probably takes place on some sort of protein framework. Eumelanin-containing melanosomes, for example, are uniformly dense and are about 1 μm in length. Phaeomelanin-containing granules on the other hand are more spherical, seem to be looser aggregates and are 2–4 nm in length. In animals that show bicoloured hair (e.g. the agouti) the base of the hair is pigmented with eumelanin with the lighter-coloured phaeomelanin at the tip.

4.4 Albinism

The condition known as *albinism* is well known and is characterized by a lack of melanin pigments. It was first described, in humans, in some American Indians in 1699, who had a milk-white skin. In fact the term covers a number of hereditary deficiency diseases, one of which is a failure to produce the enzyme tyrosinase. The condition is recessive and in addition to the lack of colour, there is a lack of daytime visual acuity and the individual experiences photophobia. As will be seen from the section on the effects of sunlight on skin (p. 37), the lack of pigmentation is quite a serious defect.

4.5 Melanocyte-stimulating hormone (MSH)

Pigmentation in animals is controlled by a hormone, MSH or *melanotropin*, produced by the anterior lobe of the pituitary. An excess of MSH produces a

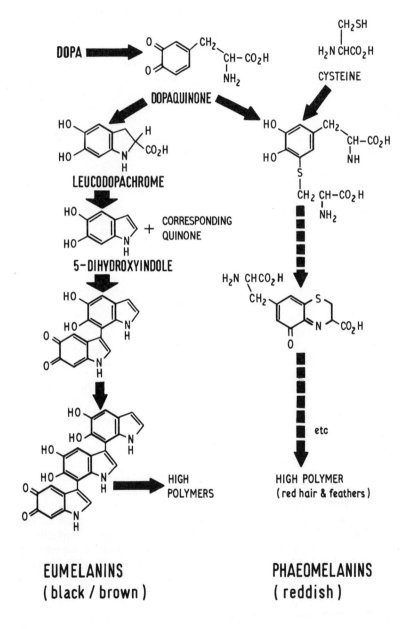

Fig. 4–2 Scheme showing the pathways of conversion of DOPA (derived from tyrosine) into eumelanins and phaeomelanins.

generalized increase in pigmentation, and the effect of MSH is to stimulate the melanocytes. The action of this hormone has been studied extensively in amphibia. When MSH is not present the melanosomes congregate near the cell nuclei and the skin then appears comparatively lightly coloured. Secretion of MSH causes the melanosomes to disperse which gives a darkening of the skin.

In humans, MSH injection causes an intense darkening of the skin over a period of 8–10 days, but the effect tends to be greater in persons with genetically dark skin to begin with. The effect seems to be to cause more melanosomes to be transferred to the keratinocytes rather than to be due to redistribution in the cell as is observed with amphibians. Moreover there is little evidence that MSH has any real role in humans. Two forms, α-MSH and β-MSH may be isolated from pituitary, the α-MSH being the most potent. However some researchers think that these may be artifacts of the isolation procedure. α-MSH is a small peptide of molecular weight about 1800 and the β-MSH is a little larger. The structure of human α-MSH (Fig. 4–3) is 13 amino acids long, and is identical with the first 13 residues of another pituitary-hormone, ACTH or adrenocorticotrophic hormone.

$$CH_3CO\text{-Ser-Tyr-Ser-Met-Glu-His-Phe-Arg-Trp-Gly-Lys-Pro-Val-}NH_2$$

Fig. 4–3 Human α-MSH. Note that the amino terminal serine residue is acetylated and that the carboxy terminal valine residue has its carboxyl group present as the amide ($-CONH_2$).

4.6 Suntan

Ultraviolet radiation is claimed to improve health, and a suntan is now equated with well being, although there is little objective evidence to support this association. Nevertheless the masses that flock to the beaches of Southern Europe every summer, as well as those using sunbeds and solaria, feel convinced that their money is well-spent and that a tan makes them sexually attractive and healthy. The immediate hazard, severe sunburn, is well known to all: a possible long-term hazard is the triggering of skin cancer. Exposure of the skin to sunlight also produces vitamin D and seems to have a positively helpful effect in some skin diseases.

4.7 Ultraviolet radiation

The ultraviolet (UV) region of the electromagnetic spectrum covers the region from 100 to 400 nm. Different wavelengths have quite different effects on skin and so it has become customary to divide the UV spectrum into three regions denoted UV-A (400–315 nm), UV-B (315–280 nm) and UV-C (280–100 nm) (Fig. 4–4). We can immediately dispose of the third region, UV-C. Rays of this wavelength are intensely damaging but fortunately do not pass through the earth's atmosphere. The UV-A region is least harmful to human skin and the main effect of light of this region is to darken a tan already

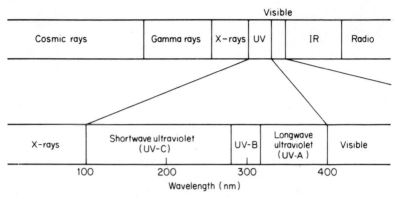

Fig. 4–4 The ultraviolet spectrum is divided into three regions, A, B and C, in terms of its effects on human skin.

initiated. However, if the skin is photosensitized, either by ingestion of certain drugs or by applying certain chemicals to the skin, then UV-A irradiation can produce reactions (see skin diseases, p. 56).

It is the narrow band of UV-B radiation that produces most of the biological effects of sun on skin, including the production of vitamin D (p. 13). UV-B radiation readily induces a tan but tends to burn first, and long-term exposure induces ageing and cancers. Sunbeds are usually designed to emit mainly UV-A. This tans slowly, but does not burn, and maintains an existing tan. However all UV lamps emit some radiation in the B and C regions, and there are dangers therefore if the source of radiation is not properly filtered.

The effects of UV-B on skin are first to produce a reddening or *erythema*. Continued exposure will lead to burning. Repeated, shortish exposures produce the desired tan, but the amount of exposure required to tan without painful or harmful burning depends on the individual, light skin being much more sensitive.

The secondary effects of UV light on skin are to produce a thickening. This, along with the increased level of melanin, protects the underlying tissues against the harmful effects of the radiation. Melanin itself is an effective absorber of UV radiation and the particles also scatter the light, diminishing its effects. Dark skins are, of course, better protected and presumably natural selection and evolution have seen to it that people of races continuously exposed to bright sunlight produce enough melanin to provide protection.

A number of preparations are now on the market which effectively screen the skin against the effects of sunlight to a greater or lesser extent. Examples of such compounds are esters of cinnamic acid and para-amino benzoic acid derivatives. Figure 4–5 shows the absorption spectra of some of these compounds and the extent to which they shield against different wavelengths. Various cosmetic agents are available which produce an artificial tan. One such agent is dihydroxyacetone which seems to react with amino acids in the skin to produce a similar colour to suntan. Such artificial tans have practically no protective effect whatever.

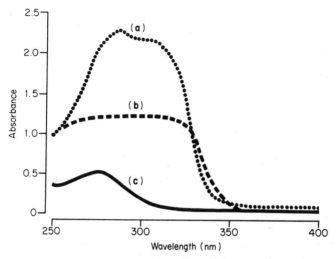

Fig. 4–5 Sunscreen preparations contain a variety of compounds which absorb in the UV-B region: (**a**) an ester of cinnamic acid; (**b**) ethyl dihydroxypropyl para-aminobenzoic acid, both spread as a layer 1 mg cm^{-2}; (**c**) stratum corneum.

Finally, in this section, brief mention must be made of the compounds called *psoralens*. These are found in certain plants and were known to the ancient Egyptians. If taken orally, the skin exhibits a sunburn response to UV-A wavelengths. One dose sensitizes for about 8 hours and in UV-A an erythema is produced and eventually a tan, without burning. This type of treatment is used in the skin disease psoriasis (see p. 60). However, it is known that psoralens bind to DNA and can prevent replication, and some medical authorities are concerned about possible long-term effects of such treatment.

4.8 Sunlight induces cancer

Cancers of the skin are most prevalent in countries such as Australia, South Africa and the southern states of the United States in which fair complexioned people are exposed to wind and more especially sun. In such countries, people of Irish and Scottish descent are particularly susceptible to sunlight-induced tumours. This has been attributed to their having developed, in their country of origin, a thin, poorly pigmented skin which may have been important in the synthesis of vitamin D at low levels of illumination.

Interestingly in the U.S.A. the incidence of skin cancer in white people of the same age group is reported to double for each 265 miles as their place of living becomes closer to the equator. In comparison, the incidence in coloured people shows only a small increase with increased exposure to sunlight. That this sort of effect is due to skin pigmentation rather than to any other factor is shown by the high incidence of skin cancer in albino Bantu. Thus the ability to tan readily without becoming sunburned seems to protect the skin by dispersing the pigment in the epidermis in a way similar to that in dark-skinned races. In sunny climates, susceptible individuals develop their skin cancers a decade or more earlier than those who tan easily.

The effect of sunlight is cumulative and the most damaging part of the spectrum is the UV-B region. It may be noted that this is largely removed by passage through glass or through water vapour and that consequently sunny, dry climates are the most dangerous.

4.9 Freckles

These are well-known and are, on the whole, not unattractive. They are probably determined by an autosomal dominant gene and are frequent in individuals with red or blond hair and blue eyes. There is no increase in the number of melanocytes in the pigmented areas or 'macules', but the melanosomes are long and rod-shaped like those found generally in the dark-skinned races. They form melanins more rapidly on exposure to sunlight than the surrounding pale skin.

It has been suggested that 'frecklers' are born with skin already occupied by two anatomically similar but functionally distinct types of melanocytes. Sunburning radiation may preferentially activate one type producing a permanent pigmented macule. Non-frecklers, who have a uniform population of melanocytes, show a uniform response to sunlight.

4.10 Porphyria

Finally in this chapter must be mentioned a group of diseases called the *porphyrias*, although they have nothing to do with melanin. The porphyrias form a group of rare, hereditary disorders in which there are defects leading to excessive production of porphyrins, the compounds that are used to form the haem in haemoglobin. These porphyrin compounds appear in the urine giving it a red colouration and their accumulation in the skin leads to acute photosensitivity. It is probable that excitation of the porphyrin by light in the presence of oxygen leads to peroxide formation and subsequent damage to the lipids of the plasma membrane and the cytoplasmic organelles. Following exposure to sunlight, erythema, oedema and vesicles appear and the photosensitivity leads to extensive ulceration of the skin and mutilating deformities, particularly on the extremities in light-exposed areas. There is hypertrichosis (excessive hair growth) in some areas, and alopecia (baldness) in others. All this, taken together with the dirty brown appearance of the teeth (which also fluoresce under a UV light) has led to the suggestion that those once known as werewolves suffered from congenital porphyria. In some forms of the disease attacks can be brought on by certain drugs, including barbiturates, sulphonamides and alcohol.

5 Inflammation, Skin Immunology and Wound Healing

5.1 Introduction

The title of this chapter covers an enormous area, a good deal of which is uncharted as far as a detailed knowledge of the multitude of processes going on is concerned. When we cut a finger we have the certainty that the cut will heal and that the skin will repair itself successfully. We little realise the complexity of the machinery involved in this everyday occurrence – inflammation and immunity to keep out infection and to clear up the debris, and cell movement and formation of new tissue to make the repair. All these processes are controlled and self-regulating so that the right things happen at the right time.

5.2 Inflammation

Many types of injurious agents give rise to an inflammatory response in the tissues of the body. These agents include mechanical, thermal or chemical trauma, bacteria and their toxins, viruses and immune reactions. All tissues show an inflammatory response but inflammation of the skin is the most obvious to us because it is visible and because the characteristic signs are immediately recognizable. These signs include redness, swelling (oedema), heat and pain and often a loss or impairment of function. Inflammation is a frequent, and indeed a normal, process as the skin performs its protective role as a barrier against the environment.

Inflammation can broadly be divided into *acute* and *chronic* types. Acute inflammation involves a succession of changes over a period of minutes to days. Chronic inflammation may last years, perhaps fluctuating in severity over this period.

The inflammatory response is a defensive reaction and involves a complicated sequence of changes. These follow a general pattern but vary in detail according to the nature of the injurious agent and the site and severity of the injury. An injury may be severe enough to cause death of cells (necrosis). Thus a burn may destroy the whole thickness of the skin, both epidermis and dermis (see Table 5–2). Dead skin cannot show inflammation, but the surrounding tissue does become inflamed and this process precedes that of wound healing (see p. 51).

The complete sequence of events in acute inflammation may be seen on a small scale when a hair follicle becomes infected with the bacterium *Staphylococcus aureus* (see p. 57). There is redness, pain and swelling and eventually an abcess (boil) develops which later discharges its purulent contents on to the skin surface. These purulent contents (pus) are a protein-containing fluid derived from plasma and may contain liquified dead tissue, dead and live white blood cells (polymorphs), and both invading and contaminating microorganisms. Such acute inflammatory events usually resolve; that is to say the signs eventually disappear and complete healing of the skin takes place.

5.3   Changes taking place in inflammation

The immediate changes taking place in inflammation are seen in the *triple response*, which occurs when a blunt point is used to draw a firm line on, say, the skin of the forearm (Fig. 5–1). First a transitory white line appears which soon becomes a red line: an initial vasoconstriction is followed by vasodilation. In the third phase, a weal develops which is an area of local swelling (oedema) and flare (irregular area of redness). The redness is caused by an increased volume of blood flowing through the inflamed area.

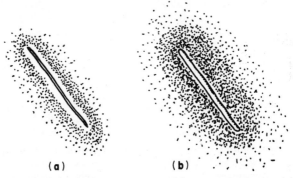

(a)   **(b)**

Fig. 5–1   The triple response. When a blunt point is drawn firmly across the skin of, say, the forearm, first a white reaction (streak) caused by vasoconstriction due to direct stimulation is seen, followed by a red reaction or flare (**a**) caused by vasodilation due to an axon reflex. After 3–5 minutes, a weal with an elevated central area due to histamine release is seen (**b**).

Two divisions of the inflammatory response can be recognized, vascular and cellular. The *vascular response* involves vasodilation, and increased vascular permeability gives rise to oedema. It is thought that the various injurious stimuli mentioned above cause the liberation of pharmacologically-active substances (Fig. 5–2) from the irritated tissues, which exert their action on blood vessels. Histamine is one of the first compounds to be released, from mast cells (see below), but its effects are short-lived. Small peptides (kinins) are mediators of the acute inflammatory response beyond the first half hour. The *cellular response* involves infiltration of granulocytes and mononuclear cells from the plasma. Normal tissues contain few extravascular polymorphs but in inflammation these cells escape from the microcirculation through the vessel wall. Chemotactic stimuli then 'guide' the cells to the site of injury: if the cells encounter bacteria and other particles then phagocytosis takes place. In this way, invading organisms and tissue debris are cleaned up, preparing the way for wound healing. The phagocytosis of bacteria and other particles can be

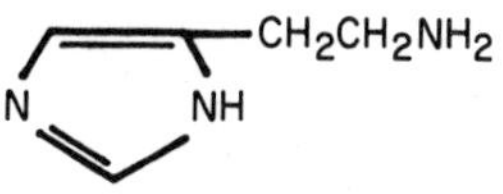

(**a**) Histamine

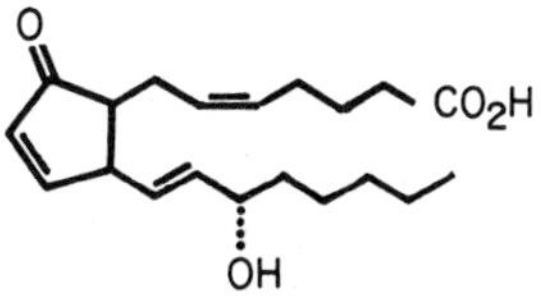

(**b**) Prostaglandin A$_2$

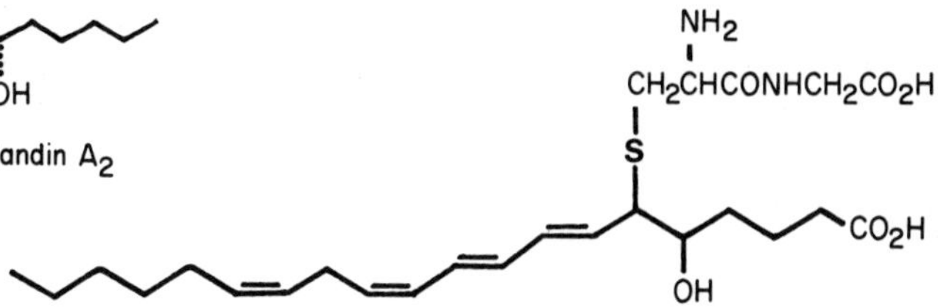

(**c**) Slow-reacting substance of anaphylaxis (SRS-A)

Fig. 5-2 Structures of some of the compounds involved in the inflammatory response. (**a**) Histamine is derived from the amino acid histidine. (**b**) Prostaglandin A$_2$, a potent arteriolar dilator, is derived from the essential fatty acid, arachidonic acid. (**c**) SRS-A is slow reacting substance of anaphylaxis. Its structure was determined in 1980 when it was shown to be a peptolipid or leukotriene, derived from arachidonic acid and the amino acids cysteine and glycine.

shown to be greatly enhanced by the presence of antibodies which are believed to coat the bacteria or foreign particles.

It has already been mentioned that inflammation may be caused by the presence of immune reactions occurring in the skin and in fact the relationship of antibodies to skin and inflammation is a very important one. In the next section we look briefly at the structure and properties of antibodies in order to set the scene for further discussion of skin immunology.

5.4 The immune system

The immune system of vertebrates is a very complex system which evolved to protect against bacterial, viral and other infections. Incidentally, it prevents organ or skin transplantation between individuals unless they are very closely related. Also when things go wrong hypersensitivity and anaphylactic shock may result.

Substances that the body recognizes as foreign ('non-self') can provoke the formation of antibodies in the blood serum. The foreign substances are referred to as *antigens* and are normally proteins or complex polysaccharides. The specific antibodies produced can combine with the antigen molecules to form an *immune complex* which can then be removed by phagocytosis in a process which normally involves the complement system (see below) as well as white cells.

The structure of antibody molecules is now very well understood and several distinct types of the antibody are recognized. All are built up on a common pattern; a basic Y-shaped structure that consists of two pairs of polypeptides. Figure 5–3 shows the structure of the IgG molecule. The sites that combine with antigen are at the ends of the arms of the Y. The stalk or tail of the Y has the property of allowing the antibody molecules (when in combination with an antigen) to be 'recognized' by other systems such as complement or phagocytic cells. Thus antibody specifically recognizes an antigen (which might for example, be a polysaccharide on the surface of a bacterium) and raises the flag to the phagocytic white cells that this is an invader to be dealt with.

The various types of antibody molecule are briefly described in Table 5–1, and each has its particular function. In relation to skin, we shall be especially interested in the type of immunoglobulin called immunoglobulin E or IgE.

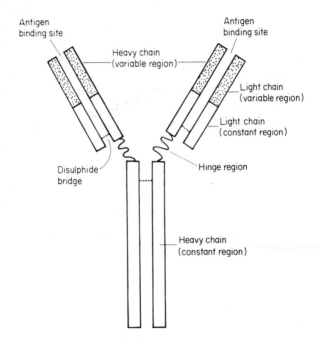

Fig. 5–3   Sketch to show the structure of the IgG molecule (diagrammatic only: in the native state the polypeptides would be coiled). The molecule is composed of four polypeptide chains, two heavy, two light, linked by disulphide bridges (dotted lines). The antigen-combining sites are at the 'top' of the arms of the 'Y' and in these regions the polypeptide chain is variable i.e. in antibody molecules of different specificities the amino acid sequences differ (stippled). The other regions of the molecule are 'constant' i.e. given types of immunoglobulin in given species have the same amino acid sequences, although these may vary in their antigen-combining properties. In the middle of the heavy chains is a more open and flexible region of polypeptide that tends to be rich in prolyl residues. Some movement of the 'amino' is possible around this so-called hinge region.

Table 5–1 Types of immunoglobulin. Five classes of immunoglobulin are found in humans and some of these have sub-classes. All are built up from the fundamental 2 heavy chain–2 light chain format, but sequences differ as does the degree of polymerization. In all, the light chains can either be κ or λ type.

Class	Heavy-chain type	Polymerization	Approx. serum concentration	Notes
IgG	γ	–	13 mg ml^{-1}	Several sub-classes known
IgM	μ	Pentamer (i.e. decavalent), plus J-chain	1 mg ml^{-1}	The first antibody to be produced in response to antigen
IgA	α	Dimers and trimers, plus secretory piece	3 mg ml^{-1}	In serum but also found in tears, saliva etc.
IgE	ϵ	–	$<1\,\mu$g ml^{-1}	Low concentration in serum but associated with mast cells. Allergy
IgD	δ	–	$<60\,\mu$g ml^{-1}	Function uncertain, ? lymphocyte surface immunoglobulin

The *complement system* of the blood is a collection of more than a dozen proteins which act in a cascade sequence when triggered off by the appropriate stimuli. Such stimuli include the presence of antibody-antigen complexes and cell-wall materials from a wide variety of microorganisms. Several consequences result from the activation of the complement system. Initially an invading organism (virus or bacterial cell) becomes coated with one of the complement proteins, marking it out to phagocytic cells as an invader to be destroyed. Also the activation of the complement system leads to proteolysis of the complement proteins themselves, and some of the small peptides produced in this process are highly inflammatory and may also have chemotactic properties, attracting white blood-cells. When the invading organism is a cell, a final consequence of complement activation can be that a mechanism, as yet poorly understood, is activated whereby the cell membrane of the invader is weakened by being punched with numerous holes. As a result cell lysis takes place and eventually the macrophages move in to clear up the debris.

Although the complement system is an important adjunct of the immune system it can also act independently. The amounts of the various complement proteins present in the blood are more or less constant and do not vary with the immune state of the individual.

5.5   IgE and mast cells

In contrast to the other immunoglobulins, IgE is normally found in miniscule amounts in human serum (e.g. <0.1 μg ml^{-1} compared with 13 mg ml^{-1} for IgG). To a great extent this prevented its discovery and characterization until comparatively recently, although its presence had long been suspected as 'reaginic antibody'. There is now intense research interest in IgE because of its association with allergy and hypersensitive states.

Although the serum concentration of IgE is usually extremely low, this concentration is raised many-fold in allergic conditions such as hay fever and asthma. However, rather than thinking of IgE as a blood antibody we should perhaps think of it as a skin antibody since most of the body's 'stock' of IgE at any one time is not free in circulation, but is bound to two types of cell: basophils in the blood and the mast cells of connective tissue and especially skin. Mast cells are polygonal or round and have a characteristic granular cytoplasm. Each mast cell has on its surface up to 40 000 binding sites for IgE molecules which presumably bind by their 'tails' or 'stalks' leaving their antigen-combining 'arms' pointing outwards.

It is uncertain whether IgE has a beneficial role to humans. There is the possibility that it may help in rejecting certain types of parasite (helminths), but for many humans at least it seems to cause nothing but trouble since it is at the root of many allergic reactions, and has a strong connection with inflammation.

5.6   Hypersensitivity

Hypersensitivity (or allergy) is the altered state of the immune system following exposure to a particular antigen. A second and subsequent contact with the same antigen may have very dramatic and serious consequences for the individual. Several types of hypersensitivity reactions are recognized, including hay fever and asthma, blood transfusion reactions, serum sickness and contact dermatitis. The reaction of the body is called *anaphylaxis* and may be so severe as to lead to death. Serum sickness, for example, used to be a common occurrence when horse antiserum was used as a protection against tetanus. A first injection of horse serum would do its job of protecting, but would *also* be recognized by the human as a foreign protein. Subsequent injections of horse serum, in some individuals, produced major anaphylactic reactions, including skin rashes, fever, swelling and joint pains.

The so-called Type I Anaphylactic reaction is that usually associated with skin reactions to drugs and to insect bites. The chain of events occurring is as follows. Antigen combines with IgE on the surface of a mast cell (or a basophil). It seems necessary for one molecule of antigen to combine with two adjacent IgE molecules, cross-linking them. When this occurs there is degranulation of the mast cell (or the basophil), with the release of histamine, kinins, and probably other substances such as the Slow Reacting Substance of Anaphylaxis (SRS-A) and prostaglandins (see Fig. 5–2). These cause vasodilation, increased capillary permeability, attraction of eosinophils to the site of reaction, and all the effects of inflammation. The cutaneous reaction is used to diagnose the hypersensitive state. This is done simply by rubbing into a scratch on the patient's skin a little of the suspected antigen.

Exactly why IgE production should be favoured in some circumstances in some individuals is not clear. Curiously, a single injection of an antigen may sometimes provoke the hypersensitive state, whereas with other antigens, prolonged contact with mucous surfaces (e.g. of grass pollen in the respiratory tract) may also lead to sensitization.

Some humans are said to be 'atopic'. Such individuals are especially prone to develop relatively high levels of IgE and hence sensitivity to 'allergens' such as pollen, house dust mites, animal dandruff, certain foods and even such drugs as penicillin. The atopic tendency, including the predeliction to asthma and hay fever, is inherited and affects as much as 10% of the population.

Serum IgE may be tested for by 'passive cutaneous anaphylaxis'. In this skin test the suspect serum is injected intradermally whereupon the IgE fixes to mast cells. Several hours later a small dose of antigen mixed with a blue dye (Evans blue) is given intravenously. If the test is positive, the reaction of antigen and IgE fixed to mast cells leads to local inflammation and increased capillary permeability which results in a visible blue patch in the skin at the site of the first injection.

Treatment of allergies includes the use of antibiotics and other drugs, with varying degrees of success. Often attempts are made to 'desensitize' the patient if the specific antigen can be detected (usually by skin patch testing). Desensitization involves injecting small, but gradually increasing amounts of the antigen (allergen). This is believed to cause a build-up of specific serum antibody (IgG), which ultimately is present in such large amounts that it tends to react with the allergen *before* it can get to the IgE attached to the mast cells in the skin.

5.7   Hypersensitivity mediated by immune complexes

When there are high levels of precipitating antibody (of any class, see Table 5–1) in the circulation, then localized injection of specific antigen can cause the formation of an antigen-antibody precipitate which is deposited in the wall of the blood vessel. In 98% of the cases these precipitates are rendered harmless by normal phagocytosis, but in a few cases there may be a serious reaction, known as *Arthus-type sensitivity*. The cutaneous response in such cases is slower (4–8 hours) than the immediate hypersensitivity reactions mentioned in the previous section, but slower than the 'delayed hypersensitivity' reaction mentioned below. The Arthus reaction is an acute inflammatory reaction with infiltration of polymorphs. The complement system may be activated and/or platelets aggregated with the release of vasoactive substances (including small peptides). The Arthus reaction is probably an exaggerated form of the normal mechanism for clearance of antigen and it is likely that it has no particular beneficial effect.

5.8   Delayed hypersensitivity

The so-called 'delayed hypersensitivity' is a cell-mediated response which gives rise to a reaction 18–48 hours after an injection of antigen. Initially a slight redness may appear at the injection site, but this gradually develops into a localized swelling. The infiltrating cells in this type of reaction are mononuclear (macrophages and lymphocytes) in contrast to the immediate type of hypersensitivity where the cellular response is mainly of polymorphonuclear leucocytes.

Delayed hypersensitivity is characteristic of infections caused by many viruses (e.g. measles, smallpox, herpes) and some bacteria (tuberculosis, brucellosis, syphilis). The skin test known as the 'tuberculin' or 'Mantoux test' is used widely in humans to discover whether the person has previously been exposed to the tubercule bacillus. In this test an intradermal extract of tubercule bacilli produces an inflammatory response appearing gradually over 18–48 hours.

Delayed hypersensitivity reactions can also result from skin contact with certain chemicals, including hair dyes, and drugs such as penicillin. These substances are themselves not antigenic but become so upon covalent binding to proteins in the skin. Clinical features of such reactions ('contact dermatitis') include redness and swelling, formation of vesicles, scaling and exudation of fluid. The nature of the mechanism by which lymphoid cells react with these materials is poorly understood.

5.9   Dermatitis

Although the skin is designed to withstand damage caused by the many and varied substances with which it comes into contact, this defence mechanism is far from perfect. This is all the more significant in our modern society where thousands of industrial chemicals are in daily use. For example, so-called irritant dermatitis accounts for 70% of industrial dermatitis. This is not associated with the induction of an allergic response, but rather results from cellular damage produced by degreasing, dehydration, denaturation of protein and upset osmotic equilibrium.

The skin's first line of defence is the surface film of emulsified sebum, sweat and cast off cells, but this is easily penetrated. The major protection is afforded by the stratum corneum. However, superficial cracking results if its water content is reduced, as happens with organic solvents and other compounds. Detergents too remove lipids and lower the water-holding capacity, causing 'chapping'. Cold air and low humidity can cause similar changes. Occlusion of the skin surface promotes percutaneous absorption and this is of great importance in individuals wearing rubber or plastic gloves, but it should not be overlooked that rings and watch-straps, as well as adhesive plasters and footwear can also have an occlusive effect. Fat-soluble substances can be absorbed via the ducts of the sebaceous and sweat glands and the hair follicles.

As with the delayed hypersensitivity reaction mentioned above the reaction produced by the skin is typically an eczematous dermatitis in which there is erythema (redness), vesicle formation, exudation and crusting. The list of chemicals that have been known to cause dermatitis (either irritant or allergic) in at least some individuals is endless. In some individuals, for example, a single immersion of the hands in a strong enzyme detergent washing powder has been known to cause acute toxic irritant dermatitis. Other substances may have a milder but more cumulative effect. Housewives, nurses, hairdressers and cleaners, lathe-workers using cutting oils, coal-miners, and workers in paint factories all come into contact with irritant chemicals. Offending substances include allyl monomers used in optical lens manufacture, trichloroethylene and methylene chloride (paint-stripper), as well as stone, coal and brick dust, fibre-glass, soap and coolants. One especially well-known example of a condition which results from exposure to organic compounds with dramatic and serious results is *chloracne*. Dioxin and other compounds such as tetrachloroazoxybenzene and chlorinated naphthalenes, are either used for, or are unwanted side-products in, the manufacture of herbicides, insecticides and wood preservatives and all can cause chloracne. This is a specific form of acne (see p. 58) in which there are numerous black comedones ('black heads') and follicular creamy spots usually occurring on the face, trunk and limbs.

If any of these toxic and irritant compounds succeeds in penetrating skin they may link with a protein which can then trigger delayed hypersensitivity and an allergic response as mentioned above. Even metals appear to be capable of doing this. Thus chrome is a common allergen in men and nickel in women and individuals in tanneries, brickworks, and in factories making anti-rusting paints and colour televisions, for example, may be affected. Other substances causing allergic dermatitis are rubber chemicals and epoxy and acrylate systems. Some of these substances can elicit a phototoxic or photoallergic response in which the pattern of eruption corresponds to the light-exposed area.

5.10   Drug reactions

Occasionally, with drugs administered to humans, there are undesirable side effects in a proportion of patients and some of these may be very serious. For example there were about 300 deaths in the U.S.A. in 1961 resulting from sensitivity to the 'life-saving' drug, penicillin. In many instances the drug reaction involves skin symptoms and it is known that these can arise by several different mechanisms, some of them immunological. An example of this is where penicillin, a small molecule that would not normally be antigenic, combines with a plasma protein. The immune system of that particular patient 'sees' this complex as a foreign protein and raises antibodies to it. If some of these antibodies are of the IgE type, then there may be a hypersensitivity reaction as described above.

Some of the types of skin reactions to drugs are given below.

(a) *Urticaria* (or hives) in which there is a transient erythema and oedema of the dermis and subcutaneous tissue. Large 'itchy' areas are formed with palpable centres but they usually disappear after 24 hours.

(b) *Purpura* which is similar to bruising and involves extravasation of red cells. Purpura can be distinguished since it does not blanch when pressed with a fingernail. Chloramphenicol and sedormid have been known to cause purpura.

(c) *Photoallergy* occurs in some drug-sensitive reactions upon exposure of the skin to light leading to eczema or urticaria. Sulphonamides and tolbutamide reaction have been known to be manifested in this way.

(d) *Exfoliative dermatitis*, with skin lesions resembling those of scarlet fever, has been observed to result, in some individuals, from the administration of barbiturates.

5.11   Viruses and the skin

Many of the hundreds of known viruses produce manifestations of disease in skin, but only a few viruses multiply *exclusively* in skin cells. Of the groups involved they seem to have few common features and indeed almost all of the major groups of virus can be involved. Many of the symptoms are of course very familiar to us in childhood diseases. To understand why the symptoms take a particular form is more difficult at our present stage of knowledge.

In measles there is a rash followed by a fine desquamation, while in chickenpox (varicella) there is a rash of papules which develop into thin-walled vesicles. The vesicular fluid becomes turbid and after 3–4 days dries up to leave a scab. Pox viruses all produce skin lesions and especially severe is smallpox in which the rash becomes papular. Soon vesicles form which become pustular and then form scabs. Herpes viruses produce vesicular eruptions especially at mucocutaneous junctions and the molluscum contagiosum virus produces small, pink, wart-like nodules on the epidermis. Finally the human wart virus (a papovirus) (p. 57) must be mentioned: the reaction of the skin is to produce a small non-malignant tumour (benign papilloma).

5.12   Transplantation immunity

At a time when heart-transplants are very frequently in the news and kidney transplantation seems almost routine, we perhaps tend to forget that much pioneering work was done many years ago with skin grafting. In any grafting or transplantation between two individuals who are not identical twins or are at least very closely related, transplant of an organ or piece of tissue will almost certainly be rejected. 'Transplantation' of blood, or blood-transfusion, is of course a highly successful procedure, although it is well understood that the blood must be of the correct 'group'. Similarly it is known that the grafting of skin from one area to another area in the same individual is successful.

Rejection of grafts between members of the same species occurs because of the existence of certain tissue antigens which are unique to the individual. These are controlled by the so-called histo-incompatibility genes which are responsible for the production of histo-incompatibility or 'transplantation' antigens (actually glycoproteins) on the cell surface. In humans the major genetic locus responsible for histocompatibility is the HL-A (for human-leukocyte-associated antigen) system which is found on the short arm of chromosome number 6. If donor and host differ in this locus, the donor tissue will be recognized as 'non-self' by the recipient's immune system and in the case of a skin graft, the grafted skin will be rejected in about 11 days. This applies to all tissues, not just skin. In order to successfully transplant between unrelated individuals, therefore, it is necessary to maintain the recipient on immunosuppressive drugs. Steroid compounds are usually given simultaneously to suppress the inflammatory response. Immunosuppressive drugs, although used very successfully, are highly dangerous ('cytotoxic') compounds, often with quite severe side effects. The danger is the greater because suppressing an individual's immune response to the transplant, simultaneously suppresses the response to any bacterial or viral infections to which the individual may be exposed. A permanent and wide-ranging antibiotic cover must therefore be given simultaneously. It can be seen that a delicate balance needs to be maintained between the various drugs for a successful transplantation.

It happens however, for reasons that are not completely understood, that despite these measures skin grafts between unrelated individuals are less easy to achieve successfully than, say, kidney transplants. For example, in an individual in which a kidney transplant is successful, a skin graft may be unsuccessful. The immunological rejection of skin grafts is in general more difficult to overcome by immunosuppression.

The actual process of rejection is mediated by the individual's cellular immune system. The *humoral immune system* is the system that produces circulating antibodies (including IgE), but there is another, or *cellular*, immune system in the body in which acquired immunity is achieved through the formation of numerous highly-specialized lymphocytes that are specifically sensitized against a foreign agent. These can attach to the foreign agent and destroy it. The class of lymphocytes responsible for the cellular response are 'T-lymphocytes' or Thymus-derived lymphocytes. Removal of the thymus before birth can completely prevent the development of all cellular immunity.

5.13   Wound healing

Tissue injury involving the skin and superficial tissues is so common that it must be looked upon as almost a 'normal' physiological process rather than a pathological one. Nevertheless an extremely complex sequence of events occurs between the acquisition of a simple cut and its repair to a mature scar. The details of the process depend to some extent on the degree of trauma suffered in the first place. Burns, for example, are classed as first, second and third degree on the amount of tissue damage (Table 5–2).

Initially there is likely to be bleeding from ruptured blood vessels as well as exudation of protein-rich fluid from the venules and capillaries bordering the injury. Quite soon the gap in the tissues becomes filled with a firm clot of blood anchored to adjacent tissues by a meshwork of the clot protein, fibrin. Two things are now necessary. First, the site must be clear of dead tissue and any infecting microorganisms and in this connection the inflammation that occurs upon wounding attracts white blood cells to the site of injury. Healing is delayed if pathogenic organisms gain access to the injured area, increasing the extent of inflammation. Second, the fibrin mesh must be replaced by strong scar tissue. A number of processes tend to be going on at the same time and it would be wrong to see them as a succession of separate events.

Within hours of injury, inflammatory cells collect in the wounded area and shortly a band of polymorphonuclear cells forms immediately below the crust of the dried clot. Repair and regeneration do not await the completion of the

Table 5–2   Classification of burns.

First-degree	Redness. Damage only to the inert surface of the skin (which will be shed and replaced). No treatment necessary.
Second-degree	Blistering. Destroys living tissue but enough of growing layer of skin left for surface to be fully restored. Closed blisters remain free from infection.
Third-degree	Involve entire thickness of skin. Loss of nerve-endings often makes 3rd-degree less painful than 1st or 2nd-degree. New skin can only grow from the edges, grafting required to cover. Scarring inevitable but skilful skin-grafting hastens recovery and reduces risk of infection.
Fourth-degree	Extensive tissue damage, charring of muscle and bone. Volume of the blood may be reduced enough to impair circulation.

Notes. Burns involving more than 10–15 per cent of the surface of the skin are likely to cause shock severe enough to require hospital treatment. In addition to the immediate damage to the tissue, blood vessels leak plasma while the blood cells remain in the blood. Failure to keep up an adequate circulation is the basis of shock.

inflammatory process however. Even while the temporary seal is forming, epidermal cells at the margin of the wound start to move into the injured area beneath the clot. In the first 24 hours the cells advance by movement alone, but after this there is an increase in epidermal mitotic activity just beyond the edge of the wounded zone. This enhanced mitotic activity, producing new cells, persists until the wound is covered (underneath the scab) with epidermis. Some time later the epidermal cells start to mature and develop a horny layer (Fig. 5–4). In spite of much work, it is still not possible to say precisely how these changes are brought about.

When the wounded area has been 're-epithelialized' in this way, the crust separates leaving new epidermis. Although this immediately starts to function as a protective barrier it is not functionally complete for quite sometime.

Lower down in the dermis repair is also going on, but this happens at a much more leisurely pace than the re-epithelialization. New connective tissue fibres are laid down along the fibrin networks formed within the wound cavity, and these gradually mature. However, it takes a considerable time for the mechanical strength of the wound (both dermal and epidermal) to regain its former strength even though it appears to be complete (Fig. 5–5). Indeed, depending upon the size of the wound, the full complement of dermal connective tissue may never be replenished as elastic fibres do not appear to reform completely. While the collagen fibrils are regenerating, the other injured dermal components are also reforming. For example, new, primitive blood vessels form which later mature, but, here again, the nerve endings may take considerably longer to reform and may never attain their original, pre-injury state.

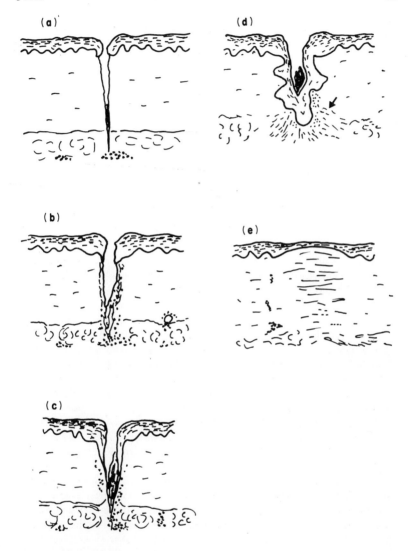

Fig. 5–4 Wound healing. Diagrammatic representation of the sequence of events in the healing of a human skin incision. (**a**) At 6 hours the epidermal margin starts to invert and there is some subcutaneous haemorrhage. (**b**) After about 2 days there is epidermal thickening, a homogeneous coagulum lines the walls of the wound and the inflammatory reaction continues. (**c**) Between 2 and 14 days epidermis starts to migrate down the walls and phagocytes are starting to remove debris. (**d**) Between 14 and 30 days epidermal proliferation continues deep into the dermis: the ridge of granulation tissue is arrowed. (**e**) After about 30 days there is a thin, raised epidermis.

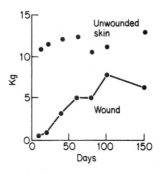

Fig. 5–5 Wound strength. Graph showing the mean tensile strength of sutured skin incision from 10–150 days compared with the strength of unwounded skin. (Redrawn from SUNDELL, B. (Ed.) (1979). *Symposium on Wound Healing*, A/S Apothekernes Laboratorium, Oslo.)

About a week after the initial injury the base of the central area of the wound, provided it is uninfected, is covered with newly formed capillaries embedded in connective tissue containing fibroblasts. There are some collagen fibres and ground substance, and macrophages and polymorphs will still be present. The lesion is red in colour and appears finely nodular or granular. The new tissue is called *granulation tissue*. Subsequently it develops and scar tissue is formed, as the inflammation dies down, in a process known as *organization*. Granulation tissue, once formed, is very resistant to infection, presumably because it is highly vascularized containing many white cells and a high concentration of antibodies. It is in the initial stages, before granulation tissue has formed, that wounds are easily infected.

Over the next week or two epithelium gradually extends over the granulation tissue. As the vascular bed is regenerating more collagen is laid down and the fibres already laid down by the fibroblasts are shortening. This draws the edges of the wound together and reduces the area which has to be re-epithelialized. After two weeks the collagen shortening will have contracted the wound and may pucker the surrounding skin. This is how a scar, or *cicatrix*, is formed and, if tissue damage has been extensive, scar contraction may severely restrict movement and incapacitate the patient. In general, the amount of scar tissue is increased in infected wounds.

The process is now nearly complete as the bright red, recently healed wound slowly transforms into an avascular white scar. Newly formed epidermis covering this is initially very thin but over a period of weeks it becomes as keratinized as the surrounding skin.

5.14 Hypertrophic scars and keloids

Sometimes, as an undesirable effect of scar formation, an excess of newly formed tissue results in the production of a hypertrophic scar. If this tissue takes on the property of unlimited growth, becoming almost a kind of tumour,

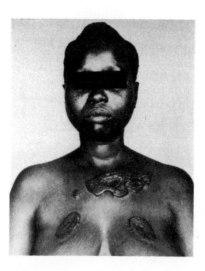

Fig. 5-6 Keloids.

it is called a *keloid*. The factors responsible for these phenomena are on the whole unknown. It is known that vertical incisions are more prone to develop in this way and there may be a genetic connection too. There seems, for example, to be an increased frequency of keloid scars in negroid races (Fig. 5–6), some of whom take advantage of the phenomenon as a form of body decoration. The excess fibrous tissue of a keloid is mostly confined to the middle and deeper layers of the dermis where there are broad interlacing bundles of collagen. Fibroblasts are present but as time passes fewer cells remain than in normal scar formation and few elastic fibres are present. The dermal appendages are lost and the overlaying epidermis becomes thinner.

6 Diseases of the Skin

6.1 Introduction

Humankind spends a great deal of money and time on its skin. An enormous cosmetics industry is devoted to enabling people to change the colour and texture of their skin and hair, to stop the sweat glands functioning and to change the natural odours of the body. A large part of the pharmaceutical industry is organized to produce creams and ointments to remove acne spots and alleviate eczema, psoriasis and other disfiguring complaints. There are many aspects to this aside from the economic ones. For example, there are the historical, social and anthropological aspects of why people paint and even disfigure their skins and of why, when they do this, people of the opposite sex find them more attractive. There is also the unavoidable moral question of the desirability of using thousands of animals each year in order to test the toxicity, to humans, of the chemicals used in the cosmetic industry. Not least, there are medical and psychological aspects, including the problems of living with a disfiguring skin condition.

There are, of course, many different forms of skin disease and the majority are not fatal. However, in a way, a disproportionate amount of time and effort is put into treating them because people tend to be very concerned that the visible parts of their bodies, namely their skins, should look 'normal' to others. Indeed just about anything wrong with the body – disease, nutritional deficiency, emotional stress – is likely to lead to some kind of visible change in the skin. Hence the concerned remark: 'You look pale today'. A healthy-looking skin is taken as a sign that the individual as a whole is healthy in body. However despite the enormous effort put into the study of skin diseases it is perhaps surprising how little is known about the root causes of the common skin diseases. In this chapter we look very briefly at some of the commonly-occurring skin complaints. In so doing the aim is not to present a gruesome catalogue of the ills that can befall humans, so much as to show how research into the biochemistry, physiology and pharmacology of the skin is slowly beginning to offer rational and effective diagnosis and treatment of skin diseases. There can be no denying, nevertheless, that there is still a long way to go.

For convenience the sections have been divided into (1) diseases caused by infection, (2) diseases of the epidermis and epidermally-derived structures, (3) diseases of the dermis, and finally, (4) cancers of the skin.

6.2 Infections

In spite of the various mechanisms to protect its surface (see p. 12), the skin does sometimes succumb to infection by viruses, bacteria, fungi and small arthropods (see p. 4). For the most part, the causes of these diseases are now quite well understood, and the treatment, for example with the appropriate antibiotic or insecticide, is usually logical, straightforward and reasonably successful.

Many virus diseases, including the common ones of childhood such as measles and chickenpox, although not solely or even directly having effects on the skin, are usually recognized by the highly characteristic pattern, colour and size of 'spots' or lesions that they produce in the skin (p. 50). Such diseases are usually encountered once or twice during childhood and are rarely encountered again, largely because, by that time, the immune system of the body has developed efficient antibodies. Others, such as cold sores (Herpes) also produce characteristic lesions but are much more difficult to get rid of because a reservoir of virus particles can exist in nervous tissue. Of the few viruses that appear to have their only effect on epidermal cells, the human wart virus (papova virus) is the most common. A wart is a small rough tumour of the epidermis, and warts are of great theoretical interest because they are the only human tumours that are certainly caused by a virus infection. A verruca is a wart on the sole of the foot. Warts often disappear spontaneously or may be 'charmed' away. A number of methods for removing warts are used, including treatment with caustics or 'keratolytic agents' (e.g. salicylic acid, podophyllum), or freezing with liquid nitrogen or solid carbon dioxide.

Of the microbial infestations of unbroken skin those caused by fungi are the commonest and also usually the most difficult to get rid of although they rarely pose a serious threat to health. *Ringworm* is an infection of the outer layer of the skin caused by a number of types of microscopic fungi belonging to the *Fungi imperfecti*, including *Trichophyton, Microsporium* and *Epidermophyton*. Often the infection spreads out to form a ring of which the centre heals, hence the name ringworm. Athlete's foot is ringworm of the feet and occurs especially between the toes. Ringworm of the scalp and the groin is particularly common, and the nails can also become infected and deformed. Itching is a natural consequence. Many forms of effective topical treatment are available but intractable cases may have to be dealt with by giving the antibiotic griseofulvin orally.

In contrast to fungal infections, pathological bacterial infections are comparatively rare on unbroken skin if we accept that it is normal to have a bacterial flora on the skin. *Impetigo* is an infection of the outer layer of the skin by the *Staphylococci*, producing clusters of small abscesses and usually irritation and scratching too. It is contagious but usually clears up upon treatment with a topical antibiotic. *Boils* are small abscesses around the roots of hairs or in sweat glands, also often caused by the staphylococci. Usually a boil is surrounded by a red, inflamed area: this is a sign that the body's defences are already at work (see p. 41). Small boils usually take care of themselves – squeezing can spread the infection. Large boils sometimes need surgically opening and/or antibiotic treatment.

Many people now apply deodorant preparations that contain antiseptics such as hexachlorophane to reduce the number of bacteria on the skin surface that break down sweat causing odour. They are rarely necessary for medical reasons and some can cause irritation and allergic rashes on sensitive skins.

6.3   Diseases of the epidermis – Acne

Acne seems to be an almost universal accompaniment of adolescence and often poses problems for the patient just at a time when he or she is acutely aware of appearance to the opposite sex. Usually it disappears at the end of the teens or by the early twenties. In adolescents however, about 15% have such serious acne that medical advice is sought. Many of the remaining 85% buy ointments and lotions 'over the counter'. The commonest form is called *acne vulgaris* and occurs mainly on the face, back and chest. Early lesions appear as non-inflamed 'blackheads' and 'whiteheads' but later each may develop an area of inflammation around it. In some cases (see Fig. 6–1) the condition is very disfiguring, and there is the possibility of permanent scarring. Acne is usually associated with a greasy skin but although dietary and psychological factors are commonly believed to cause or aggrevate acne there is little scientific evidence to support this. Indeed the true cause of acne remains unknown, although it is mainly attributed to a defect in the mechanism of action of the sebaceous glands leading to the production of large quantities of sebum. This over-production is primarily androgen-induced perhaps representing a hyper-responsiveness of the sebaceous glands to circulating androgen. Other causative factors include blockage of the pilosebaceous duct and subsequent colonization with bacteria including *Propionibacterium acnes* and *Staphylococcus epidermidis*, and the yeast *Pityrosporum ovale*. However these organisms are common on acne-free skin and are not believed to cause acne. Nevertheless, production of biologically active compounds by the bacteria obstructs the ducts and may cause inflammation.

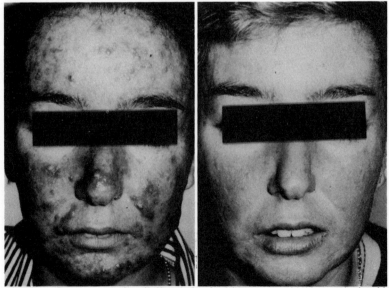

Fig. 6–1   Severe acne before (*left*) and after (*right*) treatment with 13-*cis*-retinoic acid. The photograph on the right was taken about 3½ months after treatment had commenced.

Many treatments for acne have been used. Benzoyl peroxide in a cream base is very effective in the majority of mild cases, but more severe cases should also receive oral antibiotics, such as tetracycline or erythromycin. Recently a new drug has been introduced, 13-*cis* retinoic acid, a synthetic derivative of vitamin A, which has a remarkable effect on sebaceous glands, reducing their size, and producing marked clinical improvement in severe acne (Fig. 6–1). It had been known for a long time of course that vitamin A (retinol) (Fig. 6–2), as well as having a role in the visual process, also affects epidermal differentiation. A deficiency of vitamin A in the diet leads to hyperkeratinization and mucous membrane epithelia start to keratinize. The 13-*cis* derivative of retinoic acid (Fig. 6–2) is certainly very effective but it is uncertain how it acts in acne. However the retinoid group of compounds promises to be extremely useful in other areas of dermatology (see p. 62).

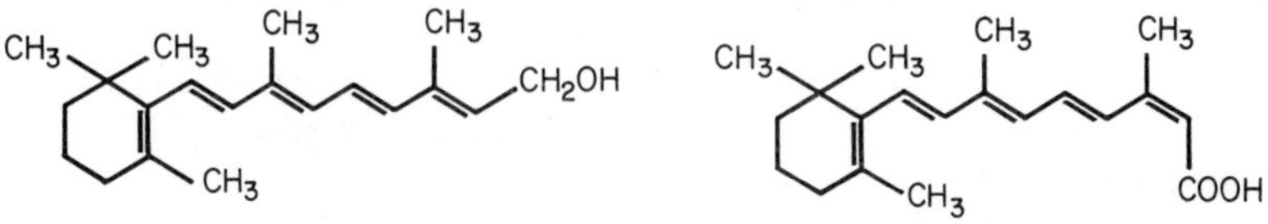

Vitamin A (Retinol)   13-*cis*-retinoic acid

Fig. 6–2   Structure of vitamin A (retinol) and 13-*cis*-retinoic acid, a drug used in the treatment of acne (see Fig. 6–1).

6.4   Eczema

Eczema, a common, non-infective inflammatory disorder of the skin, is a form of *dermatitis*. The condition affects the upper dermis and epidermis, and the symptoms are intense itching and the development of a weeping rash, with erythema (redness) and swelling (oedema). The initial change is an oedema of the lower epidermis (spongiosis) and later microscopic vesicles form. The itching causes scratching and the roofs of the vesicles tend to be rubbed off whereupon the oedema fluid leaks out. Attacks in adults are infrequent but babies often have the so-called 'infantile eczema' which they usually grow out of. Some individuals, however, develop chronic eczema in which the oedematous, parakeratotic, thickened epidermis has a characteristic appearance and 'feel' with exaggerated skin lines. This condition is called 'lichenification'.

Atopic eczema is a chronic atopic dermatitis which usually begins in infancy and is frequently associated with hay fever, asthma, or dry skin conditions. The disease probably results from any one of an assortment of disorders, most of them related in some way to allergy. Often the eczema behaves like a type of asthma, being likely to flare up without warning or at times of emotional stress. The course of the disease is unpredictable but in the long term tends to become less severe or disappear.

Seborrhoeic eczema is common in people with greasy skins and in its usual, mild form it consists of small scaly spots on the scalp with an excessive formation of dandruff. Occasionally it spreads to the ears, neck and face as a superficial scaling or a more severe eczema with exudation, crusting or thick scales. The cause is unknown and may be unrelated to the excessive sebum production. It usually responds well to simple ointments or lotions for removing scales and grease. Ordinary dandruff is a harmless scaly condition of the scalp in which the fine scales made up of the dead cells of the stratum corneum tend to accumulate.

6.5 Psoriasis

Psoriasis is a very common disorder of the outer layer of the skin, affecting between one and two percent of the population. The typical appearance is of well-defined pink or dull red blotches surmounted by a characteristic silvery scaling (Fig. 6–3). Almost any region of the skin can be involved, including the scalp, the palms and soles, and the nails, but fortunately the face is hardly ever affected even when the lesions are widespread elsewhere. There is a genetic predisposition to the disease but its cause, despite an enormous amount of medical research, remains a mystery.

Even in cases where a large part of the skin surface is involved, the general health of the patient is rarely affected, although in some forms of the disease there is an accompanying arthritis. Itching is not normally associated with the lesions and what distresses the patient more than anything is feeling disfigured and 'unclean'. Indeed in the past psoriasis has been confused with both leprosy and syphilis. However the disease is not infectious or contagious.

In histological sections through a psoriatic lesion it is seen that the granular layer is reduced or absent and there is *parakeratosis* with an increase in mitotic activity in the basal layer cells (Fig. 6–4). In the dermis there is papillary oedema and dilatation and tortuosity of the the papillary capillaries. The

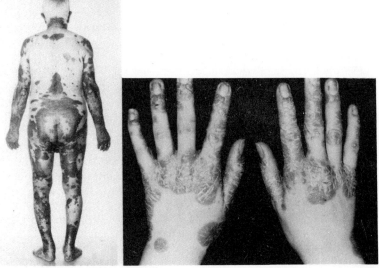

Fig. 6–3 Psoriasis: (*left*) a particularly extensive case, and (*right*) on the hands, which is rather unusual.

overall impression is that in lesions new cells are forming more quickly than dead cells are being shed from the stratum corneum.

Although the cause of the disease remains unknown, it is well established that in individuals with a genetic predisposition to the disease, certain physical and chemical trauma, infections, endocrine changes such as those occurring at puberty, certain drugs, as well as emotional stress, can all provoke the appearance of the disease or exacerbate it if it is already present. However the course of the disease is usually described as 'capricious': even without treatment it tends to come and go. With treatment it can nearly always be cleared up, at least for a time, but more often than not it returns.

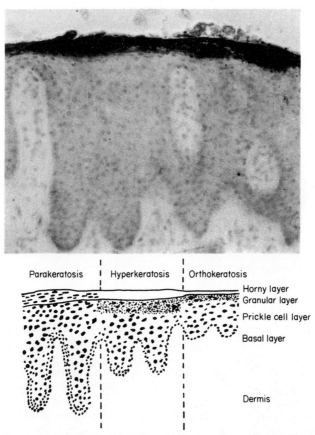

Fig. 6–4 In psoriasis there is rapid proliferation and parakeratosis. The histological section is through a psoriasis lesion: note the persistence of nuclei into the upper levels (compare Fig. 2–2). The sketch shows the difference between orthokeratosis, parakeratosis and hyperkeratosis. Orthokeratosis represents the normal situation. Nuclear remnants are retained in the horny layer only in parakeratosis. In both parakeratosis and hyperkeratosis there is thickening of the epidermis. (Redrawn from SPEARMAN, R.I.C. (1982). *The Biochemistry of Skin Disease*, Molecular Aspects of Medicine, vol. 5. Pergamon Press, Oxford.)

Many forms of treatment have been tried. Sunlight and ultraviolet radiation are generally beneficial, and in severe cases a treatment known as *photochemotherapy* may be used. In this, a patient is given a dose of a compound of the psoralen group (e.g. 8-methoxypsoralen) by mouth and shortly afterwards exposed to long wave ultraviolet light (UV-A). This treatment is called PUVA therapy and in a majority of cases is successful, at least for a time (Fig. 6–5). Various coal-tar preparations are also widely used in ointments and cream bases. It is not known how these act or which of the several hundred compounds present in coal-tar is the effective one.

In very severe psoriasis which has failed to respond to other treatments the 'antimetabolite' methotrexate is sometimes given. Some of the retinoid drugs (e.g. etretinate, see Fig. 6–5) also appear to offer beneficial results in the treatment of psoriasis.

Methotrexate

8-Methoxypsoralen

Etretinate

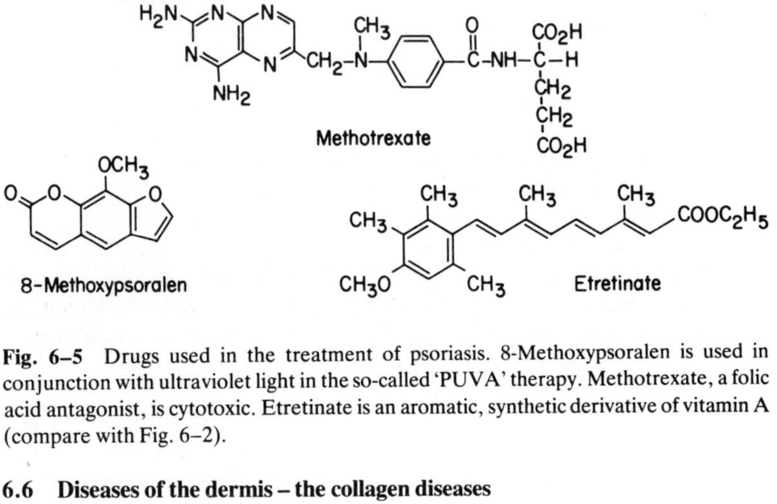

Fig. 6–5 Drugs used in the treatment of psoriasis. 8-Methoxypsoralen is used in conjunction with ultraviolet light in the so-called 'PUVA' therapy. Methotrexate, a folic acid antagonist, is cytotoxic. Etretinate is an aromatic, synthetic derivative of vitamin A (compare with Fig. 6–2).

6.6   Diseases of the dermis – the collagen diseases

A group of diseases exists, loosely known as the collagen diseases or connective-tissue diseases, which includes rheumatoid arthritis. The name is confusing since there is no evidence that collagen is primarily at fault and it seems highly likely that these are in fact *autoimmune* diseases. In this situation the immune system, which normally regards the body's own tissues as 'self' and does not make antibodies against them, goes awry and produces a sort of allergic reaction. In relation to the skin two forms of the disorder, known as *lupus erythematosus*, are the best known examples. In the first, *discoid* lupus erythematosus, there are red, often scaly patches on the skin, especially in exposed areas such as the face, and sunlight aggrevates the condition. There seems to be a genetic predisposition to the disease, associated with the possession of certain HL-A antigens, and females are more commonly affected than males. An investigation of the lesions shows liquefaction of the basal cell layer and degenerative changes in the connective tissue immediately below the epidermis. Antinuclear antibodies are present in at least a third of cases.

The condition is relatively benign. The use of sun-screens (p. 39) can help to prevent sunlight exacerbating the condition. Treatment consists of the use of topical steroid preparations or of certain compounds normally used as antimalarials (e.g. chloroquine) orally which seem to help in about 75% of cases.

In the other disease, *disseminated* lupus erythematosus, the skin changes resemble those of the discoid form, and in addition connective tissue anywhere in the body may be affected. Many of the symptoms are like those of rheumatoid arthritis. Prior to the advent of the steroid drugs, the prognosis for the patient was poor, but at the present time the use of corticosteroids, usually for a long period or even indefinitely, is life-saving.

Little is known of the cause of these diseases and future research may show (a) that they are not very closely related, and (b) that the systemic disease is in fact a group of diseases.

6.7   Diseases of collagen biosynthesis

In contrast to the diseases mentioned in the previous section, a number of diseases are known in which collagen biosynthesis and structure are deficient. These diseases can, of course, affect many of the organs of the body because collagen-containing connective tissue is widespread. However many of them produce characteristic changes in the skin. Perhaps the easiest one to understand is scurvy, caused by insufficient dietary vitamin C or ascorbic acid. The enzyme that normally adds hydroxyl groups to the amino acid residue proline in collagen (see p. 23) requires, for its activity, the presence of ferrous ion and ascorbic acid (Table 6–1). Therefore in scurvy, collagen containing insufficient hydroxyproline is formed. This collagen fails to cross-link properly and is less stable than normal collagen, which leads to increased capillary fragility and to haemorrhages, especially in the skin.

Many other diseases involving deficient collagen formation are known and are of genetic origin: many of them produce effects in the connective tissue that forms a major part of the dermis (p. 20). Most of these diseases are referred to as belonging to the Ehlers-Danlos syndrome. For example, in Type VI Ehlers-Danlos syndrome, the enzyme lysylhydroxylase is deficient or absent (Table 6–1). Consequently collagen lacking hydroxylysyl residues forms which is incapable of cross-linking. In addition to deformities in the joints, the skin of such patients shows hyperextensibility (Fig. 6–6). In Type V Ehlers-Danlos syndrome the enzyme lysyl oxidase, whose normal function is to convert the ε-amino group of lysine to an aldehyde grouping which will subsequently be used in cross-linking, is missing. Here again the presence of abnormal dermal collagen results in hyperextensibility of the skin.

6.8   Cancers of the skin

Not least amongst the diseases of the skin are cancerous diseases. These may be epithelial, melanocytic or mesodermal in origin and the study of their origin, pathology and treatment forms a very large part of the speciality of dermatology. It is only possible in the space available to offer a few remarks

Table 6–1   Enzymes involved in the formation of collagen and deficiency diseases associated with lack of them.

Prolyl hydroxylase (deficiency of ascorbic acid in scurvy lowers activity)

proline   4-hydroxyproline

Lysyl hydroxylase (scurvy, as above, and hereditary deficiency in Ehlers-Danlos syndrome type VI)

lysyl residue   hydroxylysyl residue

Lysyl oxidase (hereditary deficiency in type V Ehlers-Danlos syndrome)

lysyl (or hydroxylysyl) residue   corresponding aldehyde

---

about the incidence and epidemiology of skin cancer and to mention briefly the most commonly occurring of the diseases. The influence of sunlight, and the protective effect of melanin, has already been mentioned. In addition to sunlight, there is the possibility of developing skin tumours because of exposure to carcinogenic compounds and radiations in the environment, especially the industrial environment. In some areas the prevalence of skin cancer has been increasing over the past 10–20 years. No doubt many factors are responsible, including industrial chemicals, but changing habits of dress and the popularity of sunbathing probably also contribute.

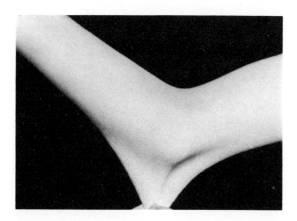

Fig. 6–6 Hyperextensibility of the skin in Ehlers-Danlos syndrome, one of the collagen diseases.

Amongst the well-recognized environmental causes are certain chemicals and this dates from the description by Potts over two centuries ago of cancer of the scrotum in chimney-sweeps. The cause of this was prolonged contact of the soot from coal fires with the scrotal skin. Since then many other environmental carcinogens have been recognized, including a number of hydrocarbons in coal-tar and various oils (mineral, creosote, cutting, as well as crude paraffin).

It is always important to decide whether tumours are benign or malignant, and whether they are of dermal or epidermal origin. The best evidence of malignancy is invasion of neighbouring tissues by atypical cells, and malignant tumours often have irregular contours whereas many benign tumours have a symmetrical shape suggestive of more or less equal growth about an axis. The determination of the origin of a tumour, dermal or epidermal, will often also determine the treatment. This is a complex area and much depends on the experience of the specialist.

6.9 Basal-cell carcinoma

This sort of cancer of the skin is also called a 'rodent ulcer' and is the commonest malignant tumour of the skin. The tumour arises from the basal area of the epidermis and is composed of cells resembling the immature cells of the epidermis, in other words the cells show little tendency either towards keratin formation or to the formation of cells characteristic of the epidermal appendages. Typically a basal cell carcinoma is slow growing, arises on the face during the later years of life, and shows little tendency to form metastases in other tissues. Men appear to be affected more frequently than women. Although the tumours are not metastatic, they do invade contiguous tissues including cartilage and bone, and as they are relatively avascular there is a tendency for them to undergo necrosis and ulceration in the central area. The lesion usually commences as a small, hard, painless nodule which enlarges slowly over a period of one and a half to three years until it becomes circular or oval, about 1 cm in diameter, and has started to undergo necrosis at the centre. Untreated, it then erodes deeper tissues and once the underlying bone is involved, it may be untreatable. However, if caught early in the development the lesions can be removed surgically or treated with radiation and the prospects are excellent.

6.10   Squamous cell carcinoma

In contrast to a basal cell carcinoma, a squamous cell carcinoma (previously called an 'epithelioma') is a tumour arising within the epidermis whose cells show a degree of maturation towards keratin formation. Most of such tumours arise as a result of some exogenous agency, including the environmental carcinogens alone or in combination, and of which sunlight is the most common. Squamous cell carcinoma develops mainly in later life (over 45) and males are affected about twice as frequently as females. Several precancerous conditions are known, including *solar keratosis*, areas of hyperkeratosis which occurs in sun-exposed fair skin, and *Bowen's disease*, a red, scaly or crusted plaque, which can become malignant and progress to form a squamous cell carcinoma. Any area of the body can be involved but obviously areas exposed to sunlight are the most susceptible.

The tumour commences as a nodule which grows fairly rapidly to form an oval or circular area raised a few millimeters above the level of the surrounding skin. Ulceration may occur and the edges of a fully formed lesion are *everted*. These malignant growths are capable of metastasizing, usually via the lymphatics. The treatment depends on the circumstances and may include local destruction, radiotherapy or surgery, or a mixture of these. In good hands all the techniques give 5 year cure rates of about 90%.

6.11   Malignant melanoma

A malignant melanoma is a malignant tumour arising in the skin from epidermal melanocytes usually from an existing cellular naevus or mole. They are rare in infants and children, unusual in young adults, and, like most cancers, affect the middle-aged and elderly predominantly. Several surveys have implicated exposure to sunlight as one of the causative factors. Most adults have at least 10–20 moles, but figures show that only about one in a million of these turns into a malignant melanoma. The first visual indication is usually a colour change in the naevus and any uniform brown lesion which acquires darker brown irregular areas or elevated nodules should be viewed with suspicion. Similarly one should be wary of any bleeding from a pigmented lesion.

Although melanomas may occur anywhere on the skin, sun-exposed areas are especially prone. The back is a frequent site in males, the legs in females. They may occur on the soles and palms, and underneath the nails. The most important therapeutic procedure for their treatment is early and adequate surgery. This usually means excision with a margin of from 3–5 cm of the surrounding clinically normal skin, and down to but not including the deep fascia. Skin grafting is almost always needed to fill the deficit.

Further Reading

ALBERTS, B., BRAY, D., LEWIS, J., RAFF, M., ROBERTS, K. and WATSON, J.D. (1983). *Molecular Biology of the Cell*. Garland Publishing, New York and London.

FRASER, R.D.B., MACRAE, T.P. and ROGERS, G.E. (1972). *Keratins: Their Composition, Structure and Biosynthesis*. Thomas, Springfield, IL.

HUME, W.J. and POTTEN, C.S. (1983). Cellular organisation in animal skin epithelium. *The Biologist*, **30**, 241–6.

MACKIE, R. (1983). *Eczema and Dermatitis*. Martin Dunitz, London.

MARKS, R. (1981). *Psoriasis*. Martin Dunitz, London.

NOBLE, W.C. and NAIDOO, J. (1979). *Microorganisms and Man*. Studies in Biology No. 111. Edward Arnold, London.

PROTA, G. and THOMBON, R.H. (1976). Melanin pigmentation in mammals. *Endeavour*, **35**, 32–8.

ROOK, A., WILKINSON, D.S. and EBLING, F.J.G. (1979). *Textbook of Dermatology*. Blackwell Scientific Publications, Oxford.

RYDER, M. (1973). *Hair*. Studies in Biology No. 41. Edward Arnold, London.

WOODHEAD-GALLOWAY, J. (1980). *Collagen: The Anatomy of a Protein*. Studies in Biology No. 117. Edward Arnold, London.

Index

Abscess 57
Acne 58
Ageing 27
Albinism 35
Allergies 47
Alopecia 17
Anaphylaxis 46, 47
Antibody structure 44
Apocrine glands 28
Arthus reaction 47
Athletes foot 57
Autoimmune antibodies 63

Baldness pattern 17
Basal cells 7, 65
Blackheads 58
Boils 41, 57
Bowen's disease 66
Burns 51

Callus 1, 8
Cancer 39, 63, 65, 66
Candida spp. 4
Chloracne 49
Cicatrix 54
Collagen 21–4, 63

Complement system 45
Cosmetics 56
Cutaneous sensibility 30
Cytotoxic drugs 51

Dandruff 59
Delayed hypersensitivity 47
Demodex follicularum 5
Dermal papillae 21
Dermatitis 48, 59
Dermatoglyphics 18
Dermis 2, 20
Desensitization 47
Desquamation 12
DOPA 35

Eczema 59
Ehlers-Danlos syndrome 63
Elastin 20, 24
Epidermal melanin unit 32
Epidermis 1, 6, 21
Epithelia 2
Epithelioma 66
Epitrichial glands 29

Eponychium 18
Erythema 38
Eumelanins 34

Fibroblasts 22, 26
Filaggrin 7, 11
Freckles 40
Fungal infections 57

Glomus bodies 28
Glycosaminoglycans 25
Gooseflesh 15
Granular layer 7
Granulation tissue 54
Ground substances 25

Hair 2, 15, 17
Hidrosis 30
Histamine 42
Histidine-rich protein 11
Histiocyte 27
HL-A system 50
Holocrine secretion 14
Horny layer 7
Hyaluronic acid 25
Hydroxyproline 23, 63
Hyperextensibility 63

Hypersensitivity 63
Hypodermis 2
Hyponychium 18

Impetigo 57
Immunoglobulins 44, 46, 49
Immunosuppressive drugs 50
Inflammation 41
Intermediate filaments 9
Involucrin 12

Keloids 55
Keratin 2, 6, 8, 10
Keratinization 6, 8, 11
Keratinocytes 4, 12
Keratolytic agents 57
Krause end bulbs 31

Langerhans cells 7
Lanugo 16
Lice 5
Lipids, epidermal 12
Lupus erythematosus 62
Lunula 18

Macrophages 27
Mantoux test 48
Mast cells 27, 46
Meissner's corpuscles 30
Melanin 4, 32–35
Melanocyte 32
Melanoma 66
Melanosomes 32
Membrane-coating granule 11

Merkel's corpuscles 31
Merocrine organ 28
Metal sensitivity 9
Methotrexate 62
Milaria 30
Moles 66

Naevus 66
Nails 18

Pacinian corpuscle 31
Parakeratosis 60
Pediculus spp. 5
Phaeomelanins 34
Phasic receptors 31
Photoallergy 49
Pigmentation 32
Pilosebaceous unit 15
Porphyria 40
Prekeratin 10
Prickly heat 30
Procollagen 22
Prostaglandins 43
Psoralens 39, 62
Psoriasis 60
Purpura 49
PUVA therapy 62

Rete ridges 21
Retinoids 59
Rodent ulcer 65
Ruffini terminals 31

Scabes 5
Scars 54
Sebaceous glands 12, 14
Sebum 2, 12, 13

Skin grafts 50, 66
Solar keratosis 66
Spiny layer 6
Squalene 13
Squames 6
Squamous corneum 6
Striae 20
Sunlight 37, 64
Sweat 2, 28, 30

Temperature control 28
Terminal differentiation 11
Tonofilaments 6
Tonic receptors 31
Transplantation immunity 52
Trichochromes 34
Triple response 42
Tyrosinase 32

Urticaria 49

Vellus hair 16
Viruses 50
Vitamin A 59
Vitamin C 23, 63
Vitamin D 1, 13

Wart virus 50, 57
Whitehead 58
Wool keratins 9
Wound-healing 41, 51–54